Legal Aspects of HIV/AIDS

A Guide for Policy and Law Reform

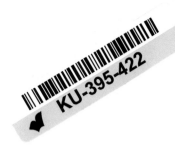

Lance Gable
Katharina Gamharter
Lawrence O. Gostin
James G. Hodge, Jr.
Rudolf V. Van Puymbroeck

Global HIV/AIDS Program
and Legal Vice Presidency
The World Bank

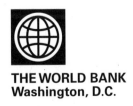

THE WORLD BANK
Washington, D.C.

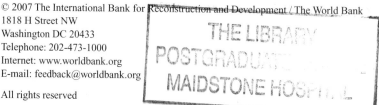
This volume is a product of the staff of the International Bank for Reconstruction and Development / The World Bank. The findings, interpretations, and conclusions expressed in this volume do not necessarily reflect the views of the Executive Directors of The World Bank or the governments they represent.

The World Bank does not guarantee the accuracy of the data included in this work. The boundaries, colors, denominations, and other information shown on any map in this work do not imply any judgement on the part of The World Bank concerning the legal status of any territory or the endorsement or acceptance of such boundaries.

Rights and Permissions

The material in this publication is copyrighted. Copying and/or transmitting portions or all of this work without permission may be a violation of applicable law. The International Bank for Reconstruction and Development / The World Bank encourages dissemination of its work and will normally grant permission to reproduce portions of the work promptly.

For permission to photocopy or reprint any part of this work, please send a request with complete information to the Copyright Clearance Center Inc., 222 Rosewood Drive, Danvers, MA 01923, USA; telephone: 978-750-8400; fax: 978-750-4470; Internet: www.copyright.com.

All other queries on rights and licenses, including subsidiary rights, should be addressed to the Office of the Publisher, The World Bank, 1818 H Street NW, Washington, DC 20433, USA; fax: 202-522-2422; e-mail: pubrights@worldbank.org.

ISBN: 978-0-8213-7105-3
eISBN: 978-0-8213-7106-0
DOI: 10.1596 / 978-0-8213-7105-3

Library of Congress Cataloging-in-Publication Data

Legal aspects of HIV/AIDS : a guide for policy and law reform / Lance Gable . . . [et al.].
    p. ; cm.
  Includes bibliographical references.
  ISBN: 978-0-8213-7105-3—ISBN: 978-0-8213-7106-0 (electronic)
  1. AIDS (Disease)—Law and legislation. 2. AIDS (Disease)—Patients—Legal status, laws, etc.
3. Public health laws. 4. Health Policy—Law and legislation. I. Gable, Lance. II. World Bank.
  [DNLM: 1. HIV Infections. 2. Health Policy—legislation & jurisprudence. 3. Health Services Accessibility—legislation & jurisprudence. 4. Public Health—legislation & jurisprudence. 5. World Health. WA 33.1 L496 2007]
  K3575.A43L436 2007
  344.04'369792—dc22

                                                                            2007023124

For more information, please contact: The Global HIV/AIDS Program, The World Bank Group, 1818 H Street, NW, Washington, DC 20433 USA; Tel: 202 458 4946; Fax: 202 522 1252; e-mail: wbglobalHIVAIDS@worldbank.org

Table of Contents

Foreword

The World Bank's Global HIV/AIDS Program of Action envisages strong World Bank support for the global response to HIV in several areas, including strengthening national strategies, accelerating implementation, and generating and sharing knowledge. This guide to the legal aspects of the pandemic ("the Guide") will help enhance the institution's contribution.

The Guide is not intended only for World Bank staff. Indeed, those who can make the best use of the information collected in this work are national AIDS councils, government ministers, and civil servants responsible for guiding and implementing their country's response to the epidemic.

Dealing successfully with HIV/AIDS cuts across almost all areas of government responsibility, and as the breadth of the 65 topics included in the Guide shows, there are many ways in which laws and regulations can either underpin or undermine good public health programs and responsible personal behaviors. The Guide indicates that statutes relating to many areas of human endeavor—from intimate private conduct to international travel—can contribute to stigma, discrimination, and exclusion or, contrariwise, can avoid and help remedy these inequities. Thus, in order to create a supportive legal framework it is important that governments identify and address effectively any gaps or other problematic aspects of their legislation and regulatory systems.

Governments are not alone in this task. Many organizations stand ready to assist and, indeed, are already doing so. A prepublication copy of the Guide was circulated to all relevant organizations of the United Nations system as well as to nongovernmental organizations and individual reviewers. Many useful suggestions for improvement have been taken into account and are gratefully acknowledged. We hope that this Guide will prove of significant, practical use to governments and their many partners in the response to HIV.

Debrework Zewdie   David Freestone
Director, Global HIV/AIDS Program   Deputy General Counsel
The World Bank   The World Bank

Acknowledgments

The Guide is the product of a team effort.

Sections 1 through 10 were principally contributed by Professors Lance Gable, Lawrence O. Gostin, and James G. Hodge, Jr., all with the Center for Law and the Public's Health at Georgetown and Johns Hopkins Universities.

Section 11 on access to medicines was principally contributed by Katharina Gamharter, Counsel/Legal Associate in the Environmentally and Socially Sustainable Development and International Law Practice Group of the World Bank's Legal Vice Presidency.

Rudolf V. Van Puymbroeck, formerly Lead Counsel for public health and HIV/AIDS in the Legal Advisory Services group of the World Bank's Legal Vice Presidency, conceived the idea, obtained the funds, found expert collaborators, contributed the section on relevant World Bank policies and procedures, and served as editor-in-chief for the work.

While we benefited from the advice and help of many, the authors would like to acknowledge in particular:

- Erin Fuse Brown, Peter Currie, Anna Dolinsky, Shira Epstein, Katie Fink, Katerina Horska, John Kraemer, Elizabeth Meltzer, Emily Stopa, and Micah Thorner for substantial research contributions to sections 1 through 10; Mark Heywood for drafting the topic on Male Circumcision; Lesley Stone for exceptional contributions to research and drafting of the sections on Injection Drug Use and Sex Work; and Katherine Razdolsky and Holly Hughes for their diligent proofreading and editorial advice.
- Fabiola Altimari, Bernard Becq, Hassane Cisse, Charles Di Leva, Alessandra Iorio, Lisa Lui, John May, Alison Micheli, Alberto Ninio, Navin Rai, Sangeeta Raja, Salman Salman, and Xinxin Yang for helpful review of, and contributions to, various topics in the section on World Bank policies and procedures. Mark Heywood, Jody Zall Kusek, Julian Fleet, Luis Gomez-Echeverr, Ralf Jürgens, Matthias Lansard, Peter McDermott and colleagues at UNICEF, Ferenc Molnar, Deena Patel, Lane Porter, and Marian Schilperoord, for their careful review and constructive suggestions for improving the Guide.
- Joy de Beyer, of the World Bank's Global HIV/AIDS Program, for handling all aspects of taking the manuscript from its first draft to final publication.
- UNAIDS for its indispensable financial support.

Explanatory Note, with Key References

The Guide is intended to be of practical use for legal reform to support effective action against HIV/AIDS. It does not aspire to provide a complete treatment of any of the 65 topics that are addressed. Rather, the Guide seeks to alert those working on AIDS strategies and projects to opportunities for legal and policy reform and to provide them with tools to tackle the job effectively. To achieve this, we adopted the following format for each topic: first, we identify the specific issue or issues raised by the topic, and we follow that with a discussion of the pertinent legal and policy considerations. Then we give at least one good practice example (often providing actual statutory language), and follow that up with a list of key references.

We realize that all of the topics could be discussed at greater length, and that a more detailed analysis of what is found in national statute books might be beneficial. However, to keep to the format of a user-friendly guide, we limited ourselves to just a few pages per topic. Hence the importance of the section on references: we count on readers who need to know more to check the sources and materials listed in the references section at the end of each topic.

That being said, there are three reference works that should be consulted first in any further research on almost any of the topics included in the Guide. Instead of repeating them 65 times, we list them here. But this is not just a measure to avoid repetition or to save paper: it is also a way of giving them the special prominence they deserve. They have been a prime source of inspiration and reference throughout the preparation of the Guide.

The first two are publications of UNAIDS, the Joint United Nations Programme on HIV/AIDS. Bringing clear human rights thinking together with sound public health policy is of fundamental importance in the field of HIV/AIDS, and these publications accomplish that admirably and consistently. The third is the product of one of the authors of the Guide. The other authors of the Guide believe that its finely honed examination of human rights considerations and public policy objectives, together with the wealth of practical experiences that it recounts, justify its inclusion in the list of basic reference sources. Here they are:

UNAIDS & Office of the United Nations High Commissioner for Human Rights, *International Guidelines on HIV/AIDS and Human Rights* (2006 Consolidated Version). http://www.unaids.org

UNAIDS & Inter-Parliamentary Union, *Handbook for Legislators on HIV/AIDS, Law, and Human Rights: Action to Combat HIV/AIDS in View of its Devastating Human, Economic, and Social Impact* (Second reprint, May 2002). http://www.unaids.org

Lawrence O. Gostin, *The AIDS Pandemic: Complacency, Injustice, and Unfulfilled Expectations* (University of North Carolina Press 2004).

About the Authors

Lance Gable, J.D., M.P.H., is Assistant Professor of Law at Wayne State University Law School and Scholar at the Center for Law and the Public's Health at Georgetown and Johns Hopkins Universities. He is co-editor (with David Buchanan and Celia Fisher) of *Ethical and Legal Issues in Research with High Risk Populations: Addressing Threats of Suicide, Child Abuse, and Violence* (forthcoming 2007), author of numerous professional journal articles, reports, and other publications, and was guest editor (with Lawrence O. Gostin and Colleen Flood) of the symposium issue *Legislating and Litigating Health Care Rights Around the World,* 33(4) J. L. Med. & Ethics (2005).

Katharina Gamharter, Dr. iur., LL.M., is Counsel/Legal Associate in the Environmentally and Socially Sustainable Development and International Law Practice Group of the World Bank's Legal Vice Presidency. She is the author of *Access to Affordable Medicines: Developing Responses under the TRIPS Agreement and EC Law* (Springer 2004) and other publications and professional journal articles related to European Union and WTO law. Previously she was Assistant Professor at the Europainstitut, Vienna University of Economics and Business Administration.

Lawrence O. Gostin, J.D., LL.D., is Associate Dean for Research and Academic Programs and Professor of Law at Georgetown University Law Center, Director of the Center for Law and the Public's Health at Georgetown and Johns Hopkins Universities, Professor of Law and Public Health at the Johns Hopkins University, Bloomberg School of Public Health, and Visiting Professor of Public Health at the Faculty of Medical Sciences, Oxford University. He is Member of the Institute of Medicine, National Academy of Sciences (lifetime), Editor (Health Law and Ethics), Journal of the American Medical Association, Co-Editor, Georgetown University Press book series, *Ethics, Health, and Public Policy,* and a member of the Editorial Board or Editorial Advisory Board of 20 professional journals. He is the author of *The AIDS Pandemic: Complacency, Injustice, and Unfulfilled Expectations* (U. of North Carolina Press 2004), and the author, co-author, or co-editor of over 30 other books or monographs as well as author or co-author of well over 100 professional journal articles in the health field.

James G. Hodge, Jr., J.D., LL.M., is Associate Professor, Johns Hopkins Bloomberg School of Public Health, Executive Director, Center for Law and the Public's Health at Georgetown and Johns Hopkins Universities, Core Faculty, Berman Bioethics Institute, Johns Hopkins Bloomberg School of Public Health, and Adjunct Faculty, Georgetown University Law Center. He teaches and lectures extensively in public health law, bioethics, and health information privacy, has authored (or co-authored) over 60 articles in professional journals and over 45 reports and other publications on public health law, bioethics, and human rights.

Rudolf V. Van Puymbroeck, J.D., M.B.A., Lic., formerly Lead Counsel, Public Health and HIV/AIDS, Legal Advisory Services, World Bank Legal Vice Presidency, is currently an independent adviser on health law and international development. He is a member of the World Bank's Editorial Committee, former member of the World Bank's Research Committee (2000–03), and co-author (with Frederick M. Abbott) of *Compulsory Licensing for Public Health: A Guide and Model Documents for Implementation of the Doha Declaration Paragraph 6 Decision* (World Bank 2005). He is former Editor of *Comprehensive Legal and Judicial Development: Toward an Agenda for a Just and Equitable Society in the 21st Century* (World Bank 2001), *The World Bank Legal Review: Law and Justice for Development* (Vol. 1, 2003), and the *Law, Justice and Development series* (World Bank 2000–03).

Acronyms

ABC	Abstain, Be faithful, and use Condoms
ADA	Americans with Disabilities Act (United States)
AIDS	Acquired Immunodeficiency Syndrome
ARV	Antiretroviral medicines/drugs
CAFTA-DR	Central America-Dominican Republic-United States Free Trade Agreement
CBO	Community-based organization
CDC	Centers for Disease Control and Prevention (United States)
CEDAW	Convention on the Elimination of All Forms of Discrimination against Women
CIOMS	Council for International Organizations of Medical Sciences
CIPIH	Commission on Intellectual Property Rights, Innovation and Public Health
COHRE	Centre on Housing Rights and Evictions
CRC	Convention on the Rights of the Child
CUP	Condom use program
DDA	Disability Discrimination Act (United Kingdom)
FC	Female circumcision (also called female genital mutilation/cutting)
FDA	U.S. Food and Drug Administration
FHI	Family Health International
FTA	Free trade agreement
FUNASA	Fundação Nacional de Saúde (National Health Foundation of Brazil)
FY	Fiscal year
HCWMP	Health Care Waste Management Plan
HIV	Human Immunodeficiency Virus

IAPSO	Inter-Agency Procurement Services Office (UNDP)
IBRD	International Bank for Reconstruction and Development
ICB	International competitive bidding
ICCPR	International Covenant on Civil and Political Rights
IDA	International Development Association
ID	Identity document
IDU	Injection/injecting drug use/user
IEDCR	Institute of Epidemiology and Disease Control
IEC	Institutional Ethics Committee
ILO	International Labour Organization
INCB	International Narcotics Control Board
IOM	International Organization for Migration
IPU	Inter-Parliamentary Union
IRBs	Institutional Review Boards
LAAM	Levo alpha acetyl methadol
LDCs	Least-developed countries (UN classification)
LGBT	Lesbian, Gay, Bisexual and Transgender
MAP	Multi-Country AIDS Program
MTCT	Mother to child transmission (of HIV)
MOH	Ministry of health
MOHP	Ministry of health and population
MSM	Men who have sex with men
MMWR RR	Morbidity and Mortality Weekly Report, Recommendations and Reports
NACOP	National AIDS Coordination Program
NEP	Needle exchange program
NGO	Nongovernment organization
NPO	Nonprofit organization
OACHA	Ontario Advisory Committee on HIV/AIDS
OHCHR	Office of the United Nations High Commissioner for Human Rights
OP/BP	Operational policy/best practice
OSI	Open Society Institute

PEP	Postexposure prophylaxis
PLHIV	Persons living with HIV
PMTCT	Prevention of mother to child transmission (of HIV)
POPs	Persistent organic pollutants
SADC/HSU	Southern African Development Community/Health Sector Unit
STD	Sexually transmitted disease
STI	Sexually transmitted infection
TB	Tuberculosis
TRIPS	Trade-Related Aspects of Intellectual Property Rights
UDHR	Universal Declaration of Human Rights
UNAIDS	Joint United Nations Programme on HIV/AIDS
UNFPA	United Nations Population Fund
UNHCHR	United Nations High Commissioner for Human Rights
UNHCR	United Nations High Commissioner for Refugees
VCT	Voluntary counseling and testing
WHO	World Health Organization
WTO	World Trade Organization

SECTION 1

Public Health Policies and Practices

1.1 Surveillance, Screening, and Testing for HIV and AIDS

The Issue

Surveillance refers to the systematic collection, analysis, interpretation, and dissemination of selected health information. HIV surveillance monitors cases of HIV infection, while AIDS surveillance tracks cases meeting the clinical definition of AIDS. Surveillance is vital to monitor the epidemic and to inform national policies. HIV testing is typically administered for individual diagnostic or clinical purposes; when it is undertaken for broader public health purposes, it is frequently referred to as screening. For example, certain populations, such as prisoners, pregnant women, and immigrants, are frequently targeted for HIV screening. Surveillance, screening, and testing all deal with sensitive personal information and raise issues of consent, privacy, and confidentiality.

Legal and Policy Considerations

Surveillance relies on test reports from public and private health settings (clinics, physicians' offices, laboratories, and nonclinical settings such as community-based organizations). There is debate over the means through which such reporting should be accomplished—whether by name, unique identifier, or anonymously. Named reporting is better able to track individual cases and to reduce duplicative reporting. But there is a trade-off between reliability of the data and facilitation of follow-up care, on the one hand, and privacy on the other. Countries need to take appropriate legal and regulatory measures to authorize the collection of HIV test data for public purposes, and to specify the reporting method and safeguard measures to be employed. In doing so, countries may find that they need to strengthen their general regulatory system for the protection of private health information.

In a joint policy statement, UNAIDS and WHO recommend distinguishing the following types of HIV testing: (1) voluntary testing (also referred to as client-initiated testing) with pre- and posttest counseling; (2) diagnostic HIV testing whenever a person shows symptoms that are consistent with HIV-related disease or AIDS; (3) routine offer of HIV testing by health care professionals for patients assessed for sexually transmitted infections, for pregnant women, and for asymptomatic people in settings where HIV is prevalent and antiretroviral treatment is available; and (4) mandatory HIV screening of all blood that is destined for transfusion or the manufacture of blood products.

Routine offer of HIV testing is referred to as opt-in testing if the person needs to give express consent before taking the test, and opt-out testing if the individual is not required to make an express statement of consent but simply retains the right to refuse the test (opting out). It should be noted that routine offer of HIV testing as set forth in the UNAIDS/WHO policy statement requires informed consent, which is defined in the policy statement as including at least the provision of information on: the clinical and prevention benefits of testing, the right to refuse, follow-up services (posttest counseling, medical care, and psychosocial support), and the importance of partner notification in the event of a positive test outcome.

In its 2006 revised recommendations for HIV testing, the U.S. Centers for Disease Control and Prevention (CDC) recommend for the United States, among other things, opt-out screening as a part of routine medical care in all health care settings, and that general informed consent for medical care be considered sufficient to encompass informed consent for HIV testing. CDC's 2001 guidelines for HIV counseling, testing, and referral include, among other things, that clients with positive test results be referred to legal services for counseling on how to prevent discrimination in employment, housing, and public accommodation.

Mandatory testing or screening involves the coercive power of the state, and should be authorized only in exceptional situations, or for narrow purposes such as blood donations. Frequently certain populations (such as immigrants, military personnel, prisoners, and persons accused or convicted of certain crimes) are subject to mandatory testing, but the professed public health benefits of these efforts tend to be illusory. In their influential handbook for legislators (see Explanatory Note, with Key References), UNAIDS and the Inter-Parliamentary Union reject such screening as a violation of human rights as well as being against good public policy.

Finally, there is anonymous HIV testing, in which no identifiable data about the person being tested is retained. Anonymous HIV testing is often guaranteed in the same laws that authorize or mandate other forms of testing. Empirical evidence suggests that the availability of anonymous testing encourages voluntary testing, particularly among members of groups who may face stigma and discrimination. Concerns about anonymous testing relate to the communication of test results, additional cost, and use for epidemiological purposes.

Practice Examples

The Quebec Public Health Act, section 33, illustrates a general surveillance provision: "Ongoing surveillance of the health status of the population and of health determinants shall be carried out so as to 1) obtain an overall picture of the health status of the population; 2) monitor trends and temporal and spatial variations; 3) detect emerging problems; 4) identify major problems; 5) develop prospective scenarios of the health status of the population; 6) monitor the development within the population of certain specific health problems and of their determinants." This provision includes surveillance for HIV infection. (Quebec *Public Health Act, R.S.Q. c. S-2.2.* http://www.canlii.org/qc/laws)

A statute providing for routine offer of HIV testing for pregnant women is the following: "As part of a health care provider's acceptance procedures or protocol, a health care provider shall provide a pregnant woman with counseling concerning being tested for the presence of HIV as part of the woman's prenatal care program. . . . The counseling shall include information that the pregnant woman does not have to consent to a test for the presence of HIV, and . . . that the pregnant woman will not be denied prenatal care by the health care provider or at the health care facility because the woman refuses to have a test performed" (Maryland Code/HEALTH-GENERAL, Sec. 18.338.2). Since a health care provider must obtain written informed consent prior to testing pursuant to Sec. 18.336 of the code, Sec. 18.338.2 is a provision for opt-in testing. (http://mlis.state.md.us)

Another example of routine testing with advance notification (opt-in) is provided by the mandatory pre-marital medical examination in France: the medical certificate must include a certification that the marriage candidate has received individual counseling on HIV and was offered an HIV test. (France, *Code de la Santé Publique, Art. L. 2121-1*)

Botswana was the first African country to move to routine opt-out screening in prenatal clinics and other health settings in 2004. (See the Rennie & Behets article and the CDC article on Botswana in the References.)

Name-based reporting of HIV-positive individuals to the Ministry of Health and Population (MOHP) is the norm in Egypt. In 2004, MOHP partnered with Family Health International to launch Egypt's first anonymous voluntary counseling and testing (VCT) site in Cairo. The availability of anonymous VCT has increased testing rates, and has provided a unique opportunity for prevention education in a country where frank discussions of sexuality and drug use are rare (FHI 2005).

The Philippines *AIDS Prevention and Control Act of 1998,* sec. 18: "The State shall provide a mechanism for anonymous HIV testing and shall guarantee anonymity and medical confidentiality in the conduct of such tests" (http://hivaidsclearinghouse.unesco.org/ev_en.php?ID=2050_201&ID2=DO_TOPIC)

In Bangladesh all medical practitioners and health care centers are required to report all AIDS cases and HIV infections to the Institute of Epidemiology and Disease Control (IEDCR). Reports are filed "using a specific form developed by IEDCR, without any identifying particulars from which the patient could be traced." (*National Policy on HIV/AIDS and STD Related Issues,* Bangladesh, 1996. http://www.ilo.org/public/english/protection/trav/aids/laws/bangladeshnationalpolicy.pdf)

References

Botswana Network on Ethics, Law, and HIV/AIDS, *Report on Routine vs. Compulsory Testing* (Botswana Network on Ethics, Law, and HIV/AIDS 2003). http://bonela.org

Csete, Joanne & Richard Elliott, *Scaling Up HIV Testing: Human Rights and Hidden Costs,* 11(1) Can. HIV/AIDS Pol. & Law Rev. (2006).

FHI, *Egypt Opens its First HIV Voluntary Counseling and Testing Site,* Insight (FHI Jan. 2005). http://www.fhi.org/NR/rdonlyres/enmw6gye5bsemdngzupd3omqdu3imaykdbn2axyuclw-jegv73o25m5uixbxc7vzgsbs7a6trjpraqg/insight7redux.pdf

————, HIV Voluntary Testing and Counseling in Egypt: A Reference Guide for Counselors. http://www.fhi.org/en/HIVAIDS/pub/res_VCTguideEgypt.htm

Jürgens, Ralf, *HIV Testing and Confidentiality: Final Report* (Canadian HIV/AIDS Legal Network & Canadian AIDS Society 2001). http://www.aidslaw.ca/publications/interfaces/downloadFile.php?ref=282

Rennie, Stuart & Frieda Behets, *Desperately Seeking Targets: The Ethics of Routine HIV Testing in Low-Income Countries*, 84(1) Bul. of the World Health Organization (2006).

UNAIDS & WHO, *UNAIDS/WHO Policy Statement on HIV Testing* (UNAIDS & World Health Organization 2004). http://data.unaids.org/una-docs/hivtestingpolicy_en.pdf

United States Centers for Disease Control and Prevention: (1) *CDC Guidelines for National Human Immunodeficiency Virus Case Surveillance, Including Monitoring for Human Immunodeficiency Virus Infection and Acquired Immunodeficiency Syndrome,* Morbidity and Mortality Weekly Report, 48, Dec. 10, 1999. (2) *Revised Guidelines for HIV Counseling, Testing and Referral,* Morbidity and Mortality Weekly Report, 50, Nov. 9, 2001. (3) *Revised Recommendations for HIV Testing of Adults, Adolescents, and Pregnant Women in Health-Care Settings*, Morbidity and Mortality Weekly Report, 55, Sept. 22, 2006. (4) *Introduction of Routine HIV Testing in Prenatal Care: Botswana, 2004,* Morbidity and Mortality Weekly Report, 53, Nov. 26, 2004.

1.2   Prevention of Mother to Child Transmission of HIV (PMTCT)

The Issue

A pregnant woman infected with HIV can transmit the virus to her fetus in the womb, during childbirth, or while breastfeeding. In the absence of intervention, the risk of mother-to-child transmission (MTCT) is 20–45%. MTCT is the most significant source of HIV infection in children below age 10. The risk of transmission can be reduced by over 40 percent by the use of antiretroviral drugs, given peripartum to the mother, or the infant, or both. In light of the clear health benefits, strong measures, sometimes of a compulsory nature, have been proposed (and enacted) for testing of pregnant women and infants, in which the interests of the child may be pitted against those of the mother.

Legal and Policy Considerations

Testing—Although the increased efficacy of antiretroviral drugs in controlling HIV infection and reducing MTCT provides a strong public health justification for widespread testing, most policy makers and health care providers oppose mandatory HIV testing for pregnant women (although many experts support routine prenatal screening). Considerations of patient autonomy are supplemented by concerns that mandatory testing may deter women from future HIV testing, prenatal care, or general medical care. Some jurisdictions do, however, impose mandatory screening on newborns if the mother does not consent to an HIV test. Policy makers and health care professionals are split on the advisability of universal screening—routine counseling and testing for all pregnant women—not just those typically considered at risk. UNAIDS, WHO, and CDC support routine offer of HIV testing to pregnant women (see Topic 1.1).

The majority of pregnant women agree to an HIV test after culturally appropriate counseling. It is important that such counseling make clear that refusal of an HIV test does not jeopardize prenatal care or legal rights. Furthermore, it should assure pregnant women that an HIV-positive result will be kept confidential (health care providers should not disclose a woman's HIV status to her spouse or partner over her objections because of the fear of domestic violence) and that it may not be used against the woman in legal proceedings, for example, to challenge child custody.

Treatment—Health care professionals, courts, and policy makers faced with a pregnant woman refusing PMTCT interventions must determine the legal and ethical balance between the adult patient's autonomy and the to-be-born child's well-being. A competent adult cannot be forced to submit to treatment for the benefit of a third person, even if that third person is her own child. But because many countries recognize the State's interest in potential life, considerations of the to-be-born child's health also raise controversial questions about the status and rights of a fetus. Studies have shown that health care providers in many high-income countries are more likely to place the interests of the fetus above those of the woman when dealing with patients from minority or low-income communities. While society recognizes a moral obligation on the part of a pregnant woman to act in the best interests of her to-be-born child, courts have typically not transformed this obligation into a legal one, especially where maximizing the welfare of the fetus involves compromising the mother's health or religious beliefs.

Practice Examples

The Constitutional Court of South Africa required the government to provide "a comprehensive and co-ordinated programme to realise progressively the rights of pregnant women and their newborn children to have access to health services to combat mother-to-child transmission of HIV . . . (which) within available resources must include reasonable measures for counselling and testing pregnant women for HIV, counselling HIV-positive pregnant women on the options open to them to reduce the risk of mother-to-child transmission of HIV, and making appropriate treatment available to them for such purposes." (Minister of Health and others v Treatment Action Campaign and others CCT 8/02, 2002 (5) SA 721 (CC) par 135. http://196.41.167.18/uhtbin/hyperion-image/J-CCT8-02A)

The CDC recommends routine opt-out HIV screening for all pregnant women as a part of antenatal care and for newborns if the mother's HIV status is unknown: "All pregnant women in the United States should be screened for HIV infection. Screening should occur after a woman is notified that HIV screening is recommended for all pregnant patients and that she will receive an HIV test as part of the routine panel of prenatal tests unless she declines (opt-out screening). HIV testing must be voluntary and free from coercion. No woman should be tested without her knowledge. Pregnant women should receive oral or written information that includes an explanation of HIV infection, a description of interventions that can reduce HIV transmission from mother to infant, and the meanings of positive and negative test results and should be offered an opportunity to ask questions and to decline testing. No additional process or written documentation of informed consent beyond what is required for other routine prenatal tests should be required for HIV testing . . . When the mother's HIV status is unknown postpartum, rapid testing of the newborn as soon as possible after birth is recommended so antiretroviral prophylaxis can be offered to HIV-exposed infants. Women should be informed that identifying HIV antibodies in the newborn indicates that the mother is infected" (CDC 2006: 9–10).

The State of New York has enacted a controversial statute for mandatory HIV testing of newborns: "In order to improve health outcomes of newborns, and to improve access to care and treatment for newborns infected with or exposed to [HIV] and their mothers, the commissioner shall establish a comprehensive program for the testing of newborns for the presence of [HIV] and/or the presence of antibodies to such virus." (NY *Public Health Law* Sec. 2500-f. http:// public.leginfo.state.ny.us)

References

National Health Committee, *HIV Screening in Pregnancy: A Report to the New Zealand Minister of Health* (National Health Committee 2004). http://www.nhc.govt.nz/publications/PDFs/hivscreening.pdf

UNAIDS, *Prevention of Mother-to-Child Transmission* (UNAIDS, accessed on 04/12/2007). http://www.unaids.org/en/Policies/HIV_Prevention/PMTCT.asp

UNAIDS & WHO, *Policy Statement on HIV Testing* (UNAIDS & World Health Organization, June 2004). http://data.unaids.org/UNA-docs/hivtestingpolicy_en.pdf

United States Centers for Disease Control and Prevention, *Revised Recommendations for HIV Testing of Adults, Adolescents, and Pregnant Women in Health-Care Settings,* Morbidity and Mortality Weekly Report, 55 (Sept. 22, 2006).

WHO, (1) *Antiretroviral Drugs for Treating Pregnant Women and Preventing HIV Infection in Infants: Towards Universal Access, Recommendations for a Public Health Approach* (World Health Organization 2006). (2) *Prevention of Mother-to-Child Transmission of HIV Infection: Generic Training Package* (World Health Organization 2004). http://www.who.int/hiv/pub/mtct/pmtct/en/index.html

————, *Pregnancy and HIV/AIDS,* Factsheet 250 (World Health Organization 2000).

Wolf, Leslie E., Bernard Lo, & Lawrence O. Gostin, *Legal Barriers to Implementing Recommendations for Universal, Routine Prenatal HIV Testing,* 32 J. L. Med. & Ethics 137 (2004).

1.3   Disclosure of HIV Information

The Issue

Disclosure of information about HIV can reveal intimate details about an individual's health status and other personal information that an individual may wish to keep private. Disclosures of HIV status can damage the privacy of persons living with HIV or AIDS and have other negative consequences such as stigma, discrimination, violence, and social isolation. Disclosure may also lead to serious economic harm, including loss of employment, insurance, or housing. On the other hand, disclosure of information about HIV may be required for public health surveillance, for the provision of appropriate medical care, and for certain nonhealth purposes such as law enforcement or insurance. Hence, countries need to develop laws and policies that balance the need for disclosure of HIV information with the protection of the privacy and autonomy of individuals with respect to their HIV status.

Legal and Policy Considerations

Privacy refers to the right of individuals to limit access by others to some aspect of their person, including health information. Privacy claims are rooted in the ethical principles of autonomy and dignity. By comparison, confidentiality extends privacy protections to special relationships, such as those between health care professionals and their patients. Privacy and confidentiality protections, as well as security measures and other laws that control the use of health data, frequently restrict the disclosure of HIV information and may provide for penalties for those who disclose HIV information without authorization or otherwise fail to comply with HIV privacy and security requirements.

The scope of limitations on disclosure of HIV test information and who is subject to these restrictions varies considerably across countries, with some countries having very robust privacy protections in place and others not providing significant privacy protections in law or practice.

A typical approach taken by many laws is to establish a default rule that the privacy of HIV information should be protected and only disclosed under specified circumstances. Beyond these specified exceptions, disclosures of HIV information, whether intentional or negligent, will constitute a breach of privacy and may result in civil liability, criminal penalties, or other serious sanctions, such as suspension of medical license.

Laws and policies that authorize disclosure of HIV information fall within three broad categories: 1) disclosures requiring informed consent; 2) discretionary disclosures; and 3) mandatory disclosures.

Requiring informed consent prior to disclosure promotes trust, cooperation, and transparency in the health care and public health systems. Informed consent also reduces the likelihood of negative consequences following the disclosure. Consent may be specific and dictate who is to receive the information, for what purposes and uses, and for how long the consent remains valid. Confidentiality laws may require additional consent for subsequent disclosures to other parties.

A second category of provisions grants individuals or institutions discretion to disclose HIV information without consent under specific circumstances outlined in law or policy. These provisions may vary greatly among countries and apply to a range of activities such as, for example, partner notification, provision of health care, court trials, or reimbursement of insurance claims. While such statutes are common, disclosures of HIV information for nonhealth purposes are controversial because they may undermine confidence in the health system, deter people from seeking testing based on privacy concerns, and may allow access to a person's HIV status in settings not governed by health information privacy laws.

The third category of authorized disclosures involves laws and policies that mandate disclosure under certain conditions. The quintessential examples of this approach are HIV reporting laws, which require physicians and laboratories to disclose positive HIV test results to the government for public health surveillance. Other examples relate to situations where there exists a duty to warn that a person may have been exposed to HIV, for example in occupational exposures or rape cases. These provisions are based on the exposed person's "right to know" about the risks they face and their need to take appropriate health protections.

Practice Examples

In the Philippines, the law applies strong confidentiality provisions to protect the privacy of HIV data. Confidentiality protections must be upheld for medical records "obtained by health professionals, health instructors, co-workers, employers, recruitment agencies, insurance companies, data encoders, and other custodians of said record, file, or data." Those who violate medical confidentiality risk imprisonment for six months to four years and other sanctions such as fines and loss of license to practice the profession. Confidential HIV test information may only be released to the person who was tested, the parent of a minor who was tested, a legal guardian of the tested person, those authorized to receive HIV information through the HIV reporting system in the government, and judges. (Philippines AIDS Prevention and Control Act of 1998: Implementing Rules and Regulations, Sec. 41–44. http://hivaidsclearinghouse.unesco.org/ ev_en.php?ID=2050_201&ID2=DO_TOPIC)

In the Ukraine, citizens have the right "to compensation for damages associated with the restriction of their rights as the result of the disclosure of information to the effect that the persons concerned are infected with HIV." (http://annualreview.law.harvard.edu/population/aids/ukraine.htm)

In a 1997 case, the European Court of Human Rights found that the publication of a person's identity and HIV status violated the person's right to respect for private and family life as guaranteed under Article 8 of the European Convention on Human Rights. (Z v. Finland, Appl. No. 22009/93, 22009/93 [1997] ECHR 10 [25 February 1997], para. 113)

In Cambodia, HIV status may be disclosed when health care professionals are complying with the country's national requirements for reporting and monitoring HIV, when HIV status needs to be disclosed in a legal setting in which the main issue is an individual's HIV status, and when "informing other health workers directly or indirectly involved in the treatment or care [of] persons with HIV/AIDS." (*Law on the Prevention and Control of HIV/AIDS,* Art. 34, Cambodia 2002. http://www.ilo.org/public/english/protection/trav/aids/laws/cambodia1.pdf)

References

AIDS Law Project & AIDS Legal Network, *Your Health Rights,* chapter 6 in *HIV/AIDS and the Law: A Resource Manual* (3rd ed., AIDS Law Project & AIDS Legal Network 2003), and App. A2 (South Africa's National Patients' Rights Charter). http://www.alp.org.za

Canadian HIV/AIDS Legal Network, *Privacy Protection and the Disclosure of Health Information: Legal Issues for People Living with HIV/AIDS in Canada* (Canadian HIV/AIDS Legal Network 2004). http://www.aidslaw.ca/publications

Center for Law and the Public's Health, *Model State Public Health Privacy Act* (Center for Law and the Public's Health). http://www.publichealthlaw.net/Resources (December 2001).

European Union, *Directive 95/46/EC of the European Parliament and of the Council of 24 October 1995 on the Protection of Individuals with Regard to the Processing of Personal Data and on the Free Movement of Such Data* (European Data Protection Directive) (European Union 1995). http://ec.europa.eu/justice_home/fsj/privacy/law/index_en.htm

Gostin, Lawrence O. & Zita Lazzarini, *Human Rights and Public Health in the AIDS Pandemic* (Oxford University Press 1997).

Jürgens, Ralf, *Confidentiality,* in *HIV Testing and Confidentiality: Final Report* (Canadian HIV/AIDS Legal Network & Canadian AIDS Society 2001). http://www.aidslaw.ca/publications/publicationsdocEN.php?ref=282

1.4   Partner Notification: The Responsibility of the Patient

The Issue

Partner notification offers a chance to increase the number of people who will seek testing and counseling for HIV, and to get more people into treatment. The partner notification process encourages (and sometimes obligates) a person to disclose his or her HIV status to sex and/or needle-sharing partners or to take efforts to reasonably protect partners from avoidable health risks. Partner notification has become a common practice around the world in HIV prevention efforts, but has remained controversial. Public health professionals justify partner notification programs as a method of prevention and access to treatment. In many cases there appears to be an ethical duty to disclose one's HIV status to partners who may be at risk of infection. This duty is grounded in the obligation to do no harm to others and the concept of a partner's "right to know" about the risks they may face. In this respect, the duty to disclose is grounded in the need to prevent further infection. Nevertheless, whether infected persons have the responsibility to inform their partners of their HIV status continues to engender debate. Some AIDS advocates argue that if a person infected with HIV consistently uses safer sex practices (using a condom), he or she may not always be obliged to inform.

Legal and Policy Considerations

In many countries, the HIV-positive index patient is primarily responsible for informing his or her sexual or needle-sharing contacts that they may have been exposed to HIV. Laws and policies have implemented this duty in the form of programs that require, or alternatively encourage on a voluntary basis, partner notification by HIV-infected individuals. In many cases, the government or other public entities will provide both the patient and partners with access to counseling, testing, and if necessary and available, treatment. Most countries that authorize partner notification prefer voluntary partner notification to other, more coercive, approaches. The UNAIDS and OHCHR *International Guidelines on HIV/AIDS and Human Rights* also adopt this approach. Likewise, UNAIDS and WHO encourage voluntary disclosure between partners and the provision of professional counseling for HIV-infected clients and their partners. Other approaches, less common, impose an affirmative duty on HIV-infected individuals to inform their partner of their HIV status on the basis of the partner's right to know. However, there likely will be situations where the patient is unable or unwilling to notify his or her partners of the risk they face. In such cases, the health care professional/counselor may be permitted to notify and counsel identified partners after weighing the harms and benefits to all parties (see Topic 1.5). Similarly, governmental public health agencies are often authorized to engage in contact tracing to identify and directly inform potential partners of the patient that they may have been exposed to HIV (see Topic 1.6).

Voluntary notification of partners can foster numerous positive outcomes, including the identification of persons potentially exposed to HIV, enabling these persons to receive counseling, testing, and if necessary, treatment; empowering partners to take appropriate precautions to avoid HIV infection or reinfection; and encourage safer behaviors in the future regardless of HIV status, which reduces further transmission of HIV.

Voluntary programs impose less on individual privacy than criminal penalties or more coercive forms of partner notification; they contribute to public awareness about HIV in the community; and may foster earlier identification of additional cases of HIV infection, opportunities to connect exposed or infected individuals to public health services, and more accurate monitoring of the HIV epidemic.

Opponents of patient-centered partner notification approaches highlight the high costs and questionable utility of partner notification as a primary strategy in reducing HIV transmission. The long incubation period of HIV may complicate the naming and location of past partners, and contacting partners raises concerns about confidentiality and stigma, particularly under partner notification laws and policies that require (not simply encourage) patients to notify partners. Partner notification carries with it the risk of domestic violence by partners who discover they may be infected with HIV. However, if HIV-infected persons do not notify their partners of their status, they may place their partners at risk for infection.

Practice Examples

In Malawi, the National AIDS Policy requires the government and its partners to promote voluntary partner notification by persons living with HIV. The government must also ensure that voluntary disclosure of HIV status is explained and encouraged during counseling and that counselors are trained to provide recommendations and assistance on how best to disclose one's HIV status to a partner (Government of Malawi, 2003).

The *Philippines AIDS Prevention and Control Act* obligates any person with HIV "to disclose his/her HIV status and health condition to his/her spouse or sexual partner at the earliest opportune time" (Philippines National AIDS Council 1998).

A study in the United States by the National Conference of State Legislatures revealed that at least 33 states have enacted HIV or AIDS-specific partner notification laws. (http://www.ncsl.org/programs/pubs/lbriefs/2001/legis642.htm)

References

Fenton, K. A. & T. A. Peterman, *HIV Partner Notification: Taking a New Look,* 11 *AIDS* 1535–46 (1997).

Gostin, Lawrence O. & James G. Hodge Jr., *Piercing the Veil of Secrecy in HIV/AIDS and Other Sexually Transmitted Diseases: Theories of Privacy and Disclosure in Partner Notification,* 1 Duke J. of Gender Law and Policy 9–88 (1998).

Government of Malawi, *National HIV/AIDS Policy: A Call for Renewed Action* (Office of the President and Cabinet, National AIDS Commission, Government of Malawi 2003). http://www.aidsmalawi.org.mw/contentdocuments

Jürgens, Ralf, *Partner Notification*, in *HIV Testing and Confidentiality: Final Report* (Canadian HIV/AIDS Legal Network & Canadian AIDS Society 2001). http://www.aidslaw.ca/publications/publicationsdocEN.php?ref=282

OACHA, *Disclosure of HIV-Positive Status to Sexual and Drug-Injecting Partners: A Resource Document* (Ontario Advisory Committee on HIV/AIDS 2003). http://www.halco.org/publications/Disclosure_Resource_Document%20Jan_03.pdf

Philippines National AIDS Council, *The Philippines AIDS Prevention and Control Act of 1998,* Sec. 34 (Philippines National AIDS Council 1998). http://hivaidsclearinghouse.unesco.org/ev_en.php?ID=2050_201&ID2=DO_TOPIC

UNAIDS, *Opening Up the HIV/AIDS Epidemic: Guidance on Encouraging Beneficial Disclosure, Ethical Partner Counseling and Appropriate Use of HIV Case-Reporting* (UNAIDS 2000). http://data.unaids.org/Publications/IRC-pub05/JC488-OpenUp_en.pdf

UNAIDS & OHCHR, *International Guidelines on HIV/AIDS and Human Rights,* 2006 Consolidated version (UNAIDS & Office of the United Nations High Commissioner for Human Rights 2006). http://data.unaids.org/Publications/IRC-pub07/JC1252-InternGuidelines_en.pdf?preview=true

WHO, *HIV Status Disclosure to Sexual Partners: Rates, Barriers and Outcomes for Women* (World Health Organization 2004). http://www.who.int/gender/documents/en/VCTinformationsheet_%5b92%20KB%5d.pdf

1.5 Partner Notification: The Duty of the Physician or Counselor

The Issue

Many countries authorize physicians or counselors to conduct partner notification. Partner notification usually is voluntary, but occasionally can be done without the consent of the index patient. A physician's duty to disclose a patient's HIV status to the patient's partners who may be at risk of infection emanates from the legal concept of "duty to warn." In order to warn the partners of an HIV-infected patient, the physician may be authorized under law to obtain the partners' names from the patient, confidentially tell the partners they may be infected, and provide the partners with HIV counseling and access to testing and other services when available. Physicians and other providers must conduct partner notification in a confidential manner to avoid violations of their patient's right to privacy and reduce possible stigma and discrimination.

Legal and Policy Considerations

In many countries, legal authority to conduct partner notification exists at multiple levels. Most countries that sanction partner notification have encouraged persons who are HIV-infected to disclose their status to partners or imposed a duty to do so (see Topic 1.4). Many of these countries have implemented additional mechanisms to authorize physicians, counselors, or other health providers to engage in partner notification when voluntary methods are insufficient or in cooperation with patients. In determining whether to employ partner notification, health care professionals must balance opposing factors. The privacy violations and potential harm, discrimination, abandonment, or stigma that the index patient may face as a result of the disclosure to partners must be weighed against the risk that, absent these efforts, HIV may be transmitted to these partners and beyond. In practice, many health care professionals avoid an active role in partner notification when patients are willing to notify their partner themselves. Only when the patient refuses or is unwilling to engage in partner notification will the physician proceed without consent. Still, a physician may determine that in light of the circumstances, such as potential abuse or other factors, partner notification may not be appropriate. Health care professionals/counselors usually retain the discretion to notify and counsel identified partners after weighing the harms and benefits to all parties.

The partner notification process may impose serious ethical dilemmas on physicians or counselors, effectively forcing them to decide between their professional obligation of confidentiality to their patient and their duty to warn the patient's partners to protect their health. Legislation that authorizes partner notification often recognizes this dilemma and provides an exception within confidentiality protections for HIV information that explicitly allows physicians to contact partners. Legislation also frequently tries to mitigate potential violations of confidentiality by requiring that physicians and counselors engaged in partner notification do not reveal the index patient's identity to notified partners. While in practice the partner may be able to determine the identity of the index patient, this process allows for the possibility of simultaneously reaching out to partners and maintaining the index patient's confidentiality.

The UNAIDS and OHCHR *International Guidelines on HIV/AIDS and Human Rights* provide important guidance on when health care professionals should engage in partner notification without consent in para. 20(g). "Public health legislation should authorize, but not require, that health-care professionals decide, on the basis of each individual case and ethical considerations, whether to inform their patients' sexual partners of the HIV status of their patient. The decision should be made in accordance with the following criteria:

  (i) the HIV-positive person in question has been thoroughly counselled;

  (ii) counselling of the HIV-positive person has failed to achieve appropriate behavioural changes;

  (iii) the HIV-positive person has refused to notify, or consent to the notification of his/her partner(s);

  (iv) a real risk of HIV transmission to the partner(s) exists;

  (v) the HIV-positive person is given reasonable advance notice;

  (vi) the identity of the HIV-positive person is concealed from the partner(s), if this is possible in practice;

  (vii) follow-up is provided to ensure support to those involved, as necessary."

Practice Examples

In Malawi, section 3.2.2.5 on "Beneficial Disclosure" of the *Policy on HIV/AIDS* permits involuntary partner notification only after "the HIV-positive person in question has been thoroughly counseled as to the need for partner notification; refused to notify or consent to the notification of his/her partner(s); a real risk of HIV transmission to an identifiable partner(s) exists; the person is given reasonable advance notice of the intention to notify; and follow-up is provided to ensure support to those involved as necessary" (Government of Malawi 2003).

Singapore employs similar provisions in its *Infectious Diseases Act* (2003).

Required vs. authorized partner notification by physicians—In Vietnam, an HIV infected person must inform his or her spouse of the infection. If the

HIV-positive person chooses not to do so, the medical establishment has to provide this information. By contrast, the New Zealand Medical Association partner notification protocol authorizes, but does not require physicians to inform and counsel partners of HIV-positive patients (see Government of Vietnam 1995).

Partner notification with or without consent—National HIV/AIDS policies in Bangladesh and Tanzania do not permit physicians to disclose HIV status to their patients' partners without the consent of the patient. Conversely, the Malawi National HIV/AIDS Policy mandates that "in exceptional cases, whereby a properly counseled HIV-positive person refused to disclose his or her status to sexual partners, the health care provider will be able to notify those partners without the consent of the source client" (see Government of Bangladesh 1996, and Government of Tanzania 2001).

References

Fenton, K. A. & T. A. Peterman, *HIV Partner Notification: Taking a New Look,* 11 *AIDS* 1535–46 (1997).

Gostin, Lawrence O. & James G. Hodge Jr., *Piercing the Veil of Secrecy in HIV/AIDS and Other Sexually Transmitted Diseases: Theories of Privacy and Disclosure in Partner Notification,* 1 Duke J. of Gender Law and Policy 9–88 (1988).

Jürgens, Ralf, *Partner Notification,* in *HIV Testing and Confidentiality: Final Report* (Canadian HIV/AIDS Legal Network & Canadian AIDS Society 2001). http://www.aidslaw.ca/Maincontent/issues/testing/11partnere.html

Government of Bangladesh, *National Policy on HIV/AIDS and STD Related Issues* (National AIDS Committee, Directorate General of Health Services, Ministry of Health and Family Welfare 1996). http://www.ilo.org/public/english/protection/trav/aids/laws/bangladeshnationalpolicy.pdf

Government of Malawi, *National HIV/AIDS Policy: A Call for Renewed Action* (Office of the President and Cabinet, National AIDS Commission, Government of Malawi 2003). www.aidsmalawi.org.mw/contentdocuments/Malawi%20National%20HIVAIDS%20Policy.pdf

Government of Singapore, *Control of AIDS and HIV Infection,* in *Infectious Diseases Act* (Government of Singapore 2003). http://agcvldb4.agc.gov.sg

Government of Tanzania, *National Policy on HIV/AIDS* (Prime Minister's Office, Government of Tanzania 2001). http://www.ilo.org/public/english/protection/trav/aids/laws/tanzanianationalpolicy.pdf

Government of Vietnam, *Ordinance on the Prevention and Fight against HIV-AIDS Infection,* 17 Official Gazette (Government of Vietnam 1995). http://www.unescap.org/esid/psis/population/database/poplaws/law_vietnam/vi014.htm

UNAIDS, *Opening Up the HIV/AIDS Epidemic: Guidance on Encouraging Beneficial Disclosure, Ethical Partner Counseling, and Appropriate Use of HIV Case-Reporting* (UNAIDS 2000). http://data.unaids.org/Publications/IRC-pub05/JC488-OpenUp_en.pdf

UNAIDS & OHCHR, *International Guidelines on HIV/AIDS and Human Rights,* 2006 Consolidated version (UNAIDS & Office of the United Nations High Commissioner for Human Rights 2006). http://data.unaids.org/Publications/IRC-pub07/JC1252-InternGuidelines_en.pdf?preview=true

1.6 Partner Notification: The Powers of Government Agencies

The Issue

In partner notification (or contact tracing), public health agencies within the government take responsibility for locating and notifying partners of HIV-infected individuals that they may have been exposed to HIV infection. Typically, the health department obtains information voluntarily from an HIV-infected person about their past and present sexual and needle-sharing partners. Health officials then use this information to trace these contacts and to notify them of their potential exposure to HIV. This process can then be repeated with new contacts. The public health justification for contact tracing differs from other types of partner notification. Rather than invoking the patient's right to know or the practitioner's duty to warn, in this context partner notification is based upon practical efforts by the public health department to prevent further infections by interrupting the chain of HIV transmission, and getting more people into treatment.

Legal and Policy Considerations

Most partner notification schemes first encourage HIV-infected patients themselves to notify their partners about their HIV status and then impose partner notification responsibility on the patient's physician or counselor if the patient is unable or unwilling to follow through with notification (see Topics 1.4, 1.5). Contact tracing often supplements these efforts or allows for some of the same results in situations in which neither of these other approaches is feasible. Some laws and policies allow physicians to refer their patients' cases to medical officers in the health department, who may have more resources than the physician to engage in partner notification.

Confidentiality is of paramount importance in the contact tracing process. Laws and policies frequently demand that public health officials take significant precautions to protect the identity of the patient who has provided contacts' information. In practice, maintaining confidentiality may be difficult as the notified contact may be able to identify the HIV-infected index patient despite the determined efforts of public health officials to maintain confidentiality. Regardless, efforts to maintain confidentiality encourage voluntary participation in partner notification efforts and reduce the likelihood of stigma, discrimination, violence, and other negative impacts associated with the disclosure of HIV status.

Partner notification can be extremely beneficial because it can offer and direct interventions to people who do not know they have been exposed to HIV. To this end, contact tracing programs should provide, whenever possible, access to HIV testing, treatment, and counseling.

Contact tracing may be expanded beyond the initial group of contacts, using information about subsequent contacts to extend HIV prevention and treatment efforts to a wider affected population. Contact tracing efforts, however, also have disadvantages. Partner notification may violate the privacy of infected patients, may be contrary to confidentiality practices applied to HIV information, may expose a person to a risk of violence when their HIV status is disclosed, and may deter people from seeking testing and treatment for HIV out of fear that their status will be disclosed to others. Another criticism of partner notification is the cost. Partner notification initiatives are relatively expensive compared to population-based HIV prevention, detection, and intervention programs. While these programs target persons who may have partnered with an infected person in the past and therefore have higher risk factors for HIV infection than the general population, the resources needed for contact, follow-up, counseling, testing, treatment, and related logistical expenses can be significant. In addition, there is considerable debate as to whether partner notification initiatives actually increase detection and reduce transmission of HIV in the population. Opponents of this approach suggest that similar results can be achieved using other public health tools—such as widespread testing, screening, counseling, and education—without raising the privacy concerns and expense of partner notification.

Practice Examples

In Mexico, the 1995 "Official Mexican Regulation for the Prevention and Control of Infection by the Human Immunodeficiency Virus" (*Norma Oficial Mexicana para la Prevención y Control de la Infección por Virus de la Immunodeficiencia Humana*) mandates the study of sexual contacts of those who are HIV-infected from the five years preceding the probable date of infection. The contact tracing investigation includes those to whom the infected person donated blood, organs, and cells, identifying those who have shared needles and syringes with the infected person, and any children potentially affected by perinatal transmission. The *Norma Oficial* stipulates that the entire investigation and any pursuit of contacts can only be done with the voluntary consent of the patient. (http://www.salud.gob.mx/unidades/cdi/nom/010ssa23.html)

Section 40 of the Philippines *AIDS Prevention and Control Act* authorizes HIV contact tracing to be pursued by the Department of Health. Information found by contact tracing must "remain confidential and classified, and can only be used for statistical and monitoring purposes." (http://hivaidsclearinghouse.unesco.org/ev_en.php?ID=2050_201&ID2=DO_TOPIC)

Several Canadian provinces have public health legislation regarding contact tracing. For example, Saskatchewan permits a designated public health officer to notify promptly all identified persons who have been exposed to a communicable disease (including HIV) without naming the source of the exposure. Physicians and nurses in the Northwest Territories are given the opportunity to request that the Chief Medical Officer carry out the contact tracing, if the physicians and nurses cannot do so on their own (see Jürgens 2001).

References

Gostin, Lawrence O. & James G. Hodge Jr., *Piercing the Veil of Secrecy in HIV/AIDS and other Sexually Transmitted Diseases: Theories of Privacy and Disclosure in Partner Notification,* 1 Duke J. of Gender Law and Policy 9–88 (1998).

Jürgens, Ralf, *Partner Notification,* in *HIV Testing and Confidentiality: Final Report* (Canadian HIV/AIDS Legal Network & Canadian AIDS Society 2001). http://www.aidslaw.ca/publications/publicationsdocEN.php?ref=282

Tapia-Conyer, Roberto, *NOM-010-SSA2-1993: Official Mexican Regulation for the Prevention and Control of Infection by the Human Immunodeficiency Virus* (Secretariat of Health, Government of Mexico 1993). http://www.salud.gob.mx/unidades/cdi/nom/010ssa23.html

1.7   Isolation and Quarantine

The Issue

Public health authorities have used isolation and quarantine to contain infectious diseases for thousands of years. These measures impose significant restrictions on movement and liberty. Isolation and quarantine may be enforced against unwilling persons who have not committed any illegal acts to protect others from the disease threat they pose. Quarantine refers to the separation and restriction of movement of persons who, while not yet ill, have been exposed to an infectious agent and therefore may become infectious. Isolation—a more relevant term in the context of HIV—involves the separation of persons known to have an infectious disease from others who are not infected, in order to reduce contact and stop the spread of illness. Isolation measures for persons infected with HIV were proposed in various settings early in the HIV epidemic, but most of these provisions were rapidly abandoned when it became clear that HIV is not transmissible through casual contact. Yet, some countries still permit individuals to be isolated due to HIV status, while others do not directly prohibit this practice.

Legal and Policy Considerations

Proposals for isolation have been based on: 1) a person's HIV-status itself, or 2) a person's propensity to engage in risky behaviors that may spread HIV. Confinement of a person solely based upon their HIV status has no public health justification. HIV can only be spread in specific ways and a status-based isolation policy would unfairly constrain the liberty of persons with HIV regardless of whether they engaged in any risky behaviors. Moreover, such a policy could be applied to restrict the movement of large numbers of people (all persons infected with HIV) for an indefinite period of time (there is no cure, so infected persons potentially could be detained for the rest of their lives). The policy would incur high costs to implement without providing any benefits to the infected and would impose stringent restrictions unnecessary to stem the spread of disease. The policy also would be a powerful deterrent to being tested for HIV, further undermining efforts to stop the spread of the disease and provide care.

Isolation based on behavioral factors is similarly unjust. Behavior-based isolation would require a finding that a particular person *might* engage in certain risky activities in the future, and would detain that person *before* he or she commits these acts. This determination would likely be highly subjective and may be applied disproportionately to minorities and those lacking political power. Predictions of future behavior are unreliable and would not be sufficient justification for a coercive measure like isolation. Isolation would also effectively prohibit persons with HIV from engaging in common voluntary activities—even consensual sexual behavior could subject a person to extended confinement.

Laws and policies should consider the specific modes of transmission of HIV and exclude isolation as an option under general communicable disease powers. Some laws explicitly prohibit the use of isolation or quarantine based on HIV status whether actual or perceived. UNAIDS and IPU suggest that if isolation absolutely must be used, it should only be employed as a last resort and for discrete periods of time for people whose behavior puts others at risk for infection. Furthermore, these organizations propose that the infected person first must be warned that if he or she does not behave responsibly, the court will take action against him or her to prevent the spread of HIV. If permitted at all, civil confinement should only proceed after a fair and impartial hearing with a guarantee of appropriate due process protections.

Practice Examples

The Philippines *AIDS Prevention and Control Act of 1998,* section 37, provides a clear prohibition on the use of isolation or quarantine in relation to HIV. "No person shall be quarantined, placed in isolation, or refused lawful entry into or deported from Philippine territory on account of his/her actual, perceived or suspected HIV status." (http://hivaidsclearinghouse.unesco.org/ev_en.php? ID=2050_201&ID2=DO_TOPIC)

When the HIV epidemic began in the 1980's, Cuba implemented a draconian policy of indefinite isolation on all known persons in the country who were infected with HIV. While there is some evidence that this limited the spread of HIV in Cuba, the use of isolation violated human rights and was widely criticized. Cuba subsequently modified this policy. HIV-infected persons in Cuba are no longer subject to indefinite isolation.

References

Gord, Cruess, *China: Alleged Quarantine of HIV Positive People in Several Provinces,* 10(2) HIV/AIDS Policy & Law Review 35 (2005).

United States Centers for Disease Control and Prevention, *Fact Sheet on Isolation and Quarantine* (United States Centers for Disease Control and Prevention 2005). http://www.cdc.gov/ncidod/sars/isolationquarantine.htm

1.8   Blood/Tissue/Organ Supply

The Issue

HIV infection can be spread through blood products, and shared human tissue and organs. The risk of infection by a transfusion of HIV-contaminated blood exceeds 90 percent. Early in the epidemic many people were infected through blood transfusions and organ or tissue donation. Once diagnostic tests were developed to detect HIV in blood and other bodily products, most countries quickly enacted laws and regulations to require screening of all blood, tissue, and organs to be used for donation in humans. Many of these laws also provide for the sanitary disposal of any sample found to be HIV-positive. Overall, these efforts have protected most transfusion and transplant recipients from receiving contaminated blood, tissue, and organ products, resulting in a substantial reduction in the incidence of HIV transmission through these products.

Legal and Policy Considerations

While it is mandatory to screen blood, tissue, and organ products for HIV around the globe, there is some variation in how this screening is done. In many places, the testing is done universally and anonymously—blood or tissues found to be infected are removed from distribution and destroyed, but the donors are not notified of their infection. Other countries have implemented systems that enable the donor to be contacted with their test results. Some countries have enforced laws that require health care professionals to suggest to those who are HIV infected that they refrain from donating blood, tissue, or organs. Additionally, some countries permit transfusion and transplantation recipients to demand a second HIV test of blood, tissue, or organ products prior to receiving them.

UNAIDS and IPU identify two vital elements for safe blood supply aside from screening blood for HIV. First, countries should have a national, nonprofit blood transfusion service that is accountable to the government. Namibia, South Africa, Zambia, and Zimbabwe, among others, all have implemented such systems. Second, blood transfusion services should take blood from voluntary donors with a low risk of infection and avoid paid or professional donors whenever possible. In Cambodia, for example, the International Committee of the Red Cross photographs blood donors who are regularly present at blood donation centers and refuses to take their blood if they are seen too often.

In several highly publicized incidents, officials and private entities in several countries were held legally responsible for neglecting to screen blood, tissue, and organ products, and thereby allowing the transmission of HIV. Many countries have made violations of blood and tissue protections punishable by law.

Countries also have created criminal penalties for misrepresenting one's HIV status on blood-donor declaration forms.

Practice Examples

WHO and UNAIDS recommend mandatory HIV screening of blood destined for transfusion or for manufacture of blood products, and bodily fluids and body parts destined for transfer or donation, such as artificial insemination, corneal grafts, and organ transplants (UNAIDS & WHO 2004).

In the Philippines, the *AIDS Prevention and Control Act of 1998* prohibits laboratories or institutions from accepting any blood, tissue, or organ donation that has not tested negative for HIV. The law provides a right to recipients of blood, tissues, or organs to demand a second HIV test on any sample, except under emergency circumstances. (http://hivaidsclearinghouse.unesco.org/ev_en.php?ID=2050_201&ID2=DO_TOPIC)

A 1998 German law regulates transfusion activities and provides rigorous testing protection for blood products. The law mandates that if a blood donation establishment detects HIV in a donor or suspects a donor of being HIV positive, the blood specimen must be removed from circulation and an inquiry must be made into the whereabouts of the donor's past donations. Under these circumstances, physicians at blood donation establishments are required to inform the donor of his or her HIV infection immediately. (http://www3.who.int/idhl-rils/frame.cfm?language=english)

In a 1996 decision, the Supreme Court of India directed the government to set up a National Blood Transfusion Council to ensure a safe blood supply, ensure all blood banks are licensed, eliminate the professional selling of blood and provide trained inspectors to check on the banks (Kumar 1996).

In the United States, Michigan mandates that every potential donor or donated specimen must be tested for HIV, and if the results of an HIV test are positive, the specimen cannot be used for transplantation, transfusion, introduction, or injection into a human body. The laws also prohibit individuals from donating blood products to a blood bank if they know that they have tested positive for HIV. (*Michigan Statutes Annotated,* sec. 333.9123, 333.11101. http://www.legislature.mi.gov/(hxesmd55osdgpvis3pwhrx45)/mileg.aspx?page=mclbasicsearch)

References

Feldman, Eric A. & Ronald Bayer, eds., *Blood Feuds: AIDS, Blood, and the Politics of Medical Disaster* (Oxford University Press 1999).

Kumar, Sanjay, *Indian Supreme Court Demands Cleaner Blood Supply,* 347 *The Lancet* 114 (1996).

Lawyers' Collective, *Legislating an Epidemic: HIV/AIDS in India,* chapter 15 (Universal Law Publishing Co. Pvt. Ltd. 2003).

Tapia-Conyer, Roberto, *NOM-010-SSA2-1993: Official Mexican Regulation for the Prevention and Control of Infection by the Human Immunodeficiency Virus* (Secretariat of Health, Government of Mexico 1993). http://www.salud.gob.mx/unidades/cdi/nom/010ssa23.html

UNAIDS, *Blood Safety and AIDS,* Best Practice Collection (UNAIDS 1997). http://data.unaids.org/Publications/IRC-pub03/Blood-PoV_en.pdf

UNAIDS & WHO, *UNAIDS/WHO Policy Statement on HIV Testing* (UNAIDS & World Health Organization 2004). http://data.unaids.org/una-docs/hivtestingpolicy_en.pdf

1.9   Universal Infection Control Precautions

The Issue

Universal infection control precautions refer to a broad set of practices intended to prevent exposure to HIV and other blood-borne pathogens in occupational or health care settings. While predominantly employed in health care settings, universal infection control precautions have also been recommended for use in other settings—for example schools, prisons, and refugee camps—where an individual may come into contact with infected blood and other bodily fluids and tissues. In health care settings, universal precautions may avert unintended HIV transmission from health care professionals to patients, from patients to health care professionals, and between patients through contaminated equipment. Transmission of HIV between patients and health care professionals can result from percutaneous injuries ("needle-stick") that expose a previously unexposed person to HIV infected blood. Patient-to-patient HIV transmission can be prevented by using new, or properly disinfected and sterilized, equipment. Other universal precautions include not recapping needles, using needles on only one patient, safely disposing of needles, using personal protective equipment such as gloves, masks, eye protection, and gowns, cleaning spills involving blood or other bodily fluids, and safely collecting and disposing of waste. Hand-washing is a very effective method of preventing transmission of a number of pathogens.

Legal and Policy Considerations

Many countries have enacted universal infection control precautions under public health legislation, regulations, or government policy. Universal precautions are recommended by numerous international organizations as well. Universal infection control precautions promote HIV prevention and reduce discrimination. The fact that the standards are applied universally allows for equal treatment in the health care system. The infection control precautions are applied to everyone without consideration of HIV status. Therefore, HIV status of health care professionals and patients becomes irrelevant for purpose of infection control and may not be used as a pretext for discrimination. Universal precautions also obviate the need for coercive HIV testing and preserve confidentiality in most circumstances. The methods used for infection control have been demonstrated to provide effective protection from occupational and health care exposures to HIV and other blood-borne agents, as well as to improve infection control throughout health care systems.

Actual implementation of universal precaution presents a challenge, particularly in lower income countries where resources for the health care system are limited. Universal precautions require support to implement, including adequate equipment, training, and education. Full and consistent application can be quite expensive, and some have argued that the cost does not justify the small number of infections that are prevented. Instead, they support enhanced precautionary measures targeted toward treating persons with HIV in health care settings and efforts to prevent HIV-infected workers from engaging in invasive procedures. Some countries have authorized exceptional precautions to be taken toward HIV infected patients or health care workers. This approach may be problematic, as patients may face discrimination or even denial of treatment based upon their perceived or actual HIV status. Furthermore, differential treatment may undermine general infection control if health care workers fail to take measures that will prevent the transmission of HIV. Some countries have not sufficiently implemented universal infection control precautions and people continue to be infected with HIV in circumstances that are easily preventable.

Practice Examples

The *Malawi National AIDS Policy,* promulgated in 2003, provides that: "Government and partners shall ensure that health care providers, home based care providers, traditional healers and traditional birth attendants are adequately trained in the application of universal precautions and are provided with the equipment necessary to implement these precautions in the course of their work. Government shall promote adherence to universal precautions to reduce the risk of HIV infection through accidental exposure to HIV and shall ensure that appropriate and accessible information on the application of universal precautions is widely disseminated." (*Malawi National AIDS Policy* sec. 3.2.2.7. http://www.ilo .org/public/english/protection/trav/aids/laws/malawinationalpolicy.pdf)

The Philippines *AIDS Prevention and Control Act of 1998, Implementing Rules and Regulations* section 21 establish "universal infection control guidelines for surgical, dental, embalming, tattooing and similar procedures." According to the Act, the universal precautions include instructions for standard hygienic procedures, especially hand-washing, disinfection and sterilization, protection of skin disease or injury with gloves or impermeable dressing, cleaning spills of blood using household bleach, wearing protective gear, and immediately disposing of needles in biohazard containers. (http://hivaidsclearinghouse .unesco.org/ev_en.php?ID=2050_201&ID2=DO_TOPIC)

The *Indonesian National Strategy of Combating AIDS* states that health care professionals must exercise universal precautions to protect themselves and their patients. The Strategy also demands delivery of training and equipment to effectively perform the necessary precautions. (*Decree No. 9/KEP/MENKO/*

KESRA/VI/ 1994 concerning the National Strategy of Combating AIDS in Indonesia. June 6, 1994. http://annualreview.law.harvard.edu/population/aids/ INDONESIA.htm)

References

SADC, *Policy Project for the SADC/HSU: National and Sector HIV/AIDS Policies in the Member States of the Southern African Development Community* (Southern African Development Community 2002). http://www.policyproject.com/pubs/countryreports/SADC.pdf

UNAIDS, *Healthcare associated infections* (UNAIDS, accessed on 04/14/2007) http://www.unaids.org/en/Policies/HIV_Prevention/Health_care_associated_infections.asp

United Nations, *Declaration of Commitment on HIV/AIDS* (United Nations General Assembly Special Session on HIV/AIDS (UNGASS), June 27, 2001). http://www.un.org/ga/aids/coverage/FinalDeclarationHIVAIDS.html

United States Centers for Disease Control and Prevention, *Universal Precautions and Creating a Safe Work Environment,* in Module 8: *Safety and Supportive Care in the Work Environment: PMTCT, Generic Training Package Trainer Manual.* (United States Centers for Disease Control and Prevention 2005). http://www.cdc.gov/nchstp/od/gap/PMTCT/Trainer%20Manual/Word/Module_8TM.doc

WHO & ILO, *Joint WHO/ILO Guidelines on Health Services and HIV* (World Health Organization & International Labour Organization 2005). http://whqlibdoc.who.int/publications/2005/9221175537_eng.pdf

1.10   Postexposure Prophylaxis

The Issue

Postexposure prophylaxis (PEP) can be an important tool to prevent HIV transmission. Available evidence suggests that prophylaxis given immediately after exposure to HIV reduces transmission rates. PEP is most commonly employed for occupational HIV exposures in health care settings (health care workers or patients exposed to HIV during treatment or while handling bodily materials) and victims of sexual assault who may be exposed to HIV by their attackers. The antiretroviral medicines used for prophylaxis can have a range of side effects of varying seriousness. Since there is urgency in the administration of PEP, the law should be clear on the rights of exposed persons and on who may be subjected to HIV testing and under what circumstances.

Legal and Policy Considerations

Laws and policies should facilitate rapid and targeted PEP for those who may have been exposed to HIV. A standard approach is to guarantee access to PEP for certain categories of possibly exposed persons, including health care workers and rape victims. Joint WHO/ILO guidelines on HIV suggest that medications for PEP (as well as voluntary, confidential counseling and testing) should be available at health service workplaces for immediate administration in the event of an exposure. Policies typically do not guarantee access to post exposure prophylaxis to other potentially exposed persons outside of these designated categories.

The debate surrounding prophylaxis policies focuses on whether PEP should be offered to all persons who potentially have been exposed to HIV, or whether PEP should only be provided if certain risk factors have been met. Since PEP should be administered very soon after the exposure, many laws and policies encourage access to PEP without first requiring HIV testing of the person or sample implicated as the source of the potential exposure. Indeed, many health experts have strongly supported the provision of universal PEP as a precautionary approach in cases where there is a high likelihood of HIV transmission and the identity—and HIV status—of the perpetrator is not known. Proposals that recommend universal PEP access for all potential HIV exposures must counsel potentially exposed persons on the side effects of the treatment, explain the risks of foregoing treatment, and account for the costs associated with post exposure prophylaxis, including drugs, HIV testing, counseling, clinical and laboratory monitoring, and serological follow-up.

Other laws and policies have sought a more targeted approach to PEP when the source of potential infection is known: first the person or sample suspected of exposing others to HIV is tested for the virus if rapid testing is available; if the test is positive, those who may have been exposed are offered immediate PEP. Voluntary testing of the source, with informed consent, is the preferred approach. However, voluntary testing of the source is not always possible. Given the severe consequences of HIV infection, some laws and policies therefore permit compelled testing of a person or sample suspected to be the source of an HIV exposure. For example, in an alleged rape situation, the law must balance the need to know the accused person's HIV status to make a more informed decision about PEP against the privacy rights of a person who has been accused—but not convicted—of a crime. Countries can avoid this dilemma by providing universal access to post exposure prophylaxis for all rape victims who may have been exposed to HIV.

Practice Examples

Many countries in southern Africa have policies regarding PEP:

The *Malawi National AIDS Policy* states (sec. 3.2.2.9): "Government and partners shall ensure access to affordable short term antiretroviral prophylaxis for persons who have experienced occupational exposure to HIV as well as to rape survivors." (http://www.aidsmalawi.org.mw/contentdocuments/Malawi%20National%20HIVAIDS%20Policy.pdf)

In Swaziland, PEP is available to health workers who are accidentally exposed to HIV. (http://www.rhap.org.za/resources/September_Pdfs/SwazilandHIV.pdf)

In South Africa, the Criminal Law (Sexual Offences and Related Matters) Amendment Bill (B50B-2006) proposes that access to PEP be part of an essential package of services available to all rape survivors.

References

de Bruyn, Theodore, *Testing of Persons Believed to be the Source of an Occupational Exposure to HBV, HCV, or HIV: A Backgrounder* (Canadian HIV/AIDS Legal Network 2001). http://www.aidslaw.ca/publications/publicationsdocEN.php?ref=288

Rey, D., M. K. Bendiane, J. P. Moatti, et al., *Post-Exposure Prophylaxis after Occupational and Non-Occupational Exposures to HIV: An Overview of the Policies Implemented in 27 European Countries,* 12(6) *AIDS Care* 695–701 (2000).

SADC, *Policy Project for the SADC/HSU: National and Sector HIV/AIDS Policies in the Member States of the Southern African Development Community* (Southern African Development Community 2002). http://www.policyproject.com/pubs/countryreports/SADC.pdf

United States Public Health Service, *Updated U.S. Public Health Services Guidelines for the Management of Occupational Exposures to HBV, HCV and HIV and Recommendations for Postexposure Prophylaxis,* 50 (RR11) Morbidity and Mortality Weekly Report 1–42 (2001).

WHO, *Post Exposure Prophylaxis* (World Health Organization, accessed on 04/12/2007). http://www.who.int/hiv/topics/prophylaxis/en/index.html (Accessed on 04/12/2007)

WHO & ILO, *Joint WHO/ILO Guidelines on Health Services and HIV* (World Health Organization & International Labour Organization 2005). http://whqlibdoc.who.int/ publications/2005/9221175537_eng.pdf

WHO & UNHCR, *Clinical Management of Rape Survivors: Developing Protocols for Use with Refugees and Internally Displaced Persons* (Revised ed., World Health Organization & United Nations High Commissioner for Refugees 2004). http://www.who.int/reproductive-health/publications/clinical_mngt_survivors_of_rape/clinical_mngt_survivors_of_rape.pf

Zungu-Dirwayi, Nompumelelo, Olive Shisana, Eric Udjo, et al., *An Audit of HIV/AIDS Policies in Botswana, Lesotho, Mozambique, South Africa, Swaziland and Zimbabwe* (Human Sciences Research Council 2004). http://www.hsrcpublishers.ac.za/index.asp?id=1926

1.11   Access to the Technical Means of Prevention (Condoms)

The Issue

Condom use is a critical element in a comprehensive, effective, and sustainable approach to HIV prevention. High quality, low cost condoms are effective as a barrier to contracting HIV. Research has shown that proper and consistent condom use greatly reduces the risk of HIV transmission. Laws have been enacted to ensure wide accessibility of condoms in sites such as night clubs, restaurants, airports and other transport stations, bathrooms, dormitories, supermarkets, pharmacies, and workplaces. Pervasive marketing and use of condoms complements other HIV prevention programs including family planning and reproductive health clinics, abstinence programs, and monogamy campaigns. Other distribution methods, such as mail order, internet order, and vending machines have the additional value of protecting the anonymity of condom buyers. However, some countries continue to perpetuate laws and policies that undermine access, use, and education about condoms.

Legal and Policy Considerations

National laws and policies around the world have recognized the importance of condoms to prevent HIV. For condoms to be safe and effective, they must be manufactured to the high international standards and quality assurance procedures established by WHO, UNFPA, and UNAIDS. Many countries have enacted laws and policies that guarantee quality standards for condoms. Furthermore, condoms must be universally readily available at either low or no cost, as this greatly increases the likelihood that they will be used. Some countries have taken steps to provide free condoms and sexual health education to specific population subgroups perceived to be at high risk for HIV transmission through sexual intercourse, such as sex workers. For condoms to succeed as a prevention tactic, they must be accompanied by education. Many countries have included education initiatives with their plans to distribute condoms. For example, Namibia's *National Strategic Plan on HIV/AIDS* includes two education initiatives related to its condom programs. These initiatives include information leaflets on how to properly put on and use a condom and training of local people to demonstrate the use of condoms to others.

Condom access may be limited by resource allocation decisions that fund other HIV prevention activities but not condoms. These decisions may respond to limitations dictated by international or national funders. Some countries prohibit adolescents from purchasing condoms without parental permission. Carrying condoms may be stigmatizing and is criminalized in certain countries. Due to the association of prostitution with condoms, legislation in some countries prohibits condom possession and forbids efforts to educate sex workers on the use of condoms to reduce HIV transmission. When the use of condoms is criminalized or used as evidence of illegal sex work, sex workers become fearful of using them and consequently have sex without protection. In 1999, under China's *State Advertisement Law,* the government banned all advertisements promoting public awareness and the use of condoms. China has since reversed course and now strongly promotes condom use, education, and access (see practice example below). Other countries have demonstrated reluctance to officially sanction condom use to prevent HIV transmission based upon religious or moral traditions that resist public discussion of sexual activities or forbid prophylaxis. A few countries have moved in the opposite direction, requiring in law that sex workers use condoms during sexual intercourse (see Topic 5.5). Finally, regardless of legislative factors involving condom access and education, the ability to use condoms is greatly impacted by social and cultural norms. In many societies, women may not be empowered to protect themselves by insisting that their partners use condoms (see Chapter 7). Therefore, protecting women's rights can create conditions in which condoms can be used more consistently and more effectively. The promotion and provision of female condoms can foster empowerment of women. Given that no effective microbicide has been developed yet, the female condom provides a unique prevention option that can be initiated by women themselves.

Practice Examples

In 2004, the Chinese Ministry of Health and other government departments issued guidelines on the distribution of condoms that emphasized HIV prevention and distribution of condoms by the health and family planning network. Further, the Ministry of Health agreed to provide free condoms to people living with HIV. On January 29, 2006, China's State Council adopted the *Regulations on the Prevention and Treatment of AIDS*, requiring operators of public entertainment venues to offer condoms or install condom vending machines. (http://www.casy.org/chron/poilcy.htm)

India's *National AIDS Prevention and Control Policy* stated that there should be no moral, ethical, or religious inhibition regarding the use of condoms. With extremely widespread distribution of condoms, the Policy states that the government will promote development of culturally acceptable information packages about condoms (Government of India 2001).

Many southern African countries have policies or strategies to increase accessibility of condoms and educate the population about condom use. Uganda's "ABC" campaign, urging residents to "Abstain, Be faithful, and use Condoms" proved effective in reducing HIV transmission rates. The Namibian government, through the National AIDS Co-ordination Program (NACOP), distributes condoms to health services, government sectors, NGOs, private companies, and higher learning institutions free of charge. Kenya's *National Condom Policy and Strategy* is an extensive document on how, when, where, and by whom condoms will be distributed and promoted. Mozambique and Malawi also have implemented major condom distribution efforts under their national HIV policies (see references).

The Argentinean government passed an ordinance on AIDS prevention requiring the installation of condom vending machines in public areas in Buenos Aires. The machines are to display instructions on how to use condoms and how to prevent HIV infection. (http://www3.who.int/idhl-rils/frame.cfm?language= english)

References

China AIDS Survey, *China HIV/AIDS Policy and Regulations Chronology* (China AIDS Survey 2004). http://www.casy.org/chron/poilcy.htm

Government of India, *National AIDS Prevention and Control Policy* (Government of India 2001). http://unpan1.un.org/intradoc/groups/public/documents/APCITY/UNPAN009846 .pdf

Government of Kenya, *National Condom Policy and Strategy: 2001–2005* (Ministry of Health & National AIDS Control Council, Republic of Kenya 2001). http://www.policyproject .com/pubs/countryreports/Kenya_Condom_Policy.pdf

Government of Namibia, *National Strategic Plan on HIV/AIDS (Medium Term Plan II), 1999–2004* (Ministry of Health and Social Services, Republic of Namibia 1999). http://hivaidsclearinghouse.unesco.org/ev_en.php?ID=3160_201&ID2=DO_TOPIC

Jayasuriya, D. C., *A Comparative Review of AIDS Legislation in Asia and the Pacific,* 43(2) Inter. and Comp. Law Q. 391–405 (1994).

UNAIDS, WHO & UNFPA, *Position Statement on Condoms and HIV Prevention* (UNAIDS, World Health Organization & United Nations Population Fund 2004). http://www.unfpa .org/upload/lib_pub_file/343_filename_Condom_statement.pdf

University of Pretoria, *HIV/AIDS and Human Rights in Namibia,* in *HIV/AIDS and Human Rights in SADC* (Center for the Study of AIDS & Center for Human Rights, University of Pretoria 2004).

————, *HIV/AIDS and Human Rights in Mozambique,* in *HIV/AIDS and Human Rights in SADC* (Center for the Study of AIDS & Center for Human Rights, University of Pretoria 2004).

————, *HIV/AIDS and Human Rights in Malawi,* in *HIV/AIDS and Human Rights in SADC* (Center for the Study of AIDS & Center for Human Rights, University of Pretoria 2004).

WHO, *Argentina (Buenos Aires). Ordinance No. 51.189 of 5 December 1996,* in *International Digest of Health Legislation* (World Health Organization 1995). http://www.who.int/idhl/

Zeldin, Wendy, *Health Law and Regulation: China, AIDS Regulations,* Global Legal Monitor, May, 25 (2006).

1.12   Male Circumcision

The Issue

Male circumcision has been carried out for religious and cultural reasons for thousands of years. Observational studies had noted significantly lower rates of HIV infection in countries and regions where the practice of male circumcision is widespread. In 2005 and 2006 three randomized controlled trials evaluated the impact of male circumcision on the risk of HIV infection in males. All three trials confirmed that male circumcision, performed by well trained medical professionals, is safe and reduced the risk of HIV infection by between 50 and 60%. Some experts estimate that if male circumcision is widely and properly carried out it could have a major impact on HIV prevalence and prevent tens of thousands of new HIV infections. It is likely that there will be a growing demand for safe, affordable male circumcision, particularly in high HIV prevalence areas. Already a number of governments in sub-Saharan Africa, led by Swaziland and Kenya, have reacted positively to the research findings, making it probable that they will introduce policies, regulations, and laws that promote and provide male circumcision.

Legal and Policy Considerations

In March 2007, information from the trials led to the WHO and UNAIDS issuing a first set of guidelines on male circumcision as an HIV prevention intervention. Whilst finding "that the efficacy of male circumcision in reducing female to male transmission of HIV has been proven beyond reasonable doubt," the guidelines are correctly cautious. They stress that male circumcision is *not* completely efficacious; that there is no evidence yet that it reduces the risk of an HIV infected man infecting a female partner; and that the risk of the creation of a false sense of security needs to be actively countered in HIV prevention and public health messaging.

> "Male circumcision should never replace other known methods of HIV prevention and should always be considered as part of a comprehensive HIV prevention package, which includes: promoting delay in the onset of sexual relations, abstinence from penetrative sex and reduction in the number of sexual partners; providing and promoting correct and consistent use of male and female condoms; providing HIV testing and counselling services; and providing services for the treatment of sexually transmitted infections."

WHO and UNAIDS advise that

> "countries considering the introduction or expansion of male circumcision services should ensure that appropriate laws, regulations and policies are developed so that male circumcision services are accessible, provided safely and without discrimination."

The Guidelines raise a number of specific legal and policy considerations. Some issues are likely to vary from country to country depending on whether there is already a widespread practice of male circumcision; who conducts it (traditional or religious health practitioners or medical doctors); and at what age male circumcision takes place (soon after birth, at adolescence, or as a rite of passage into manhood).

These issues can be summarized as:

- Ensuring safety of male circumcision and that health facilities are properly equipped, hygienic and staff appropriately trained.
- Ensuring informed consent of the person undergoing male circumcision, meaning that he is counseled on the benefits and risks, and particularly the need to continue to practice safer sex after the operation.
- Preventing the coercion of boys or men into male circumcision.
- Preventing discrimination against those who opt for or against male circumcision.
- Promoting the right of communities (not just men) "to clear and comprehensive information about what is known and not known about male circumcision."
- Promoting the right of men who chose male circumcision "to receive full information on the benefits and risks of the procedure."

In addition the Guidelines draw attention to the need to always act in the best interests of the child and to involve the male child in decision making and to seek his assent or consent to the procedure "according to his evolving capacity."

Practice Examples

The practice of male circumcision varies greatly across countries. In many countries its practice is governed by the general ethical and procedural guidelines of the medical profession, particularly guidelines that aim to ensure safety and consent for all surgical procedures. Occasionally, for example in Britain and the United States, specific professional ethical guidelines have been developed.

Male circumcision may also be governed by jurisprudence that may have developed around issues such as informed consent, medical negligence, and delict (tort). In a number of developing countries, policy makers and health officials should be aware of legislation that may have been passed either to prevent children from being coerced into circumcision, or to improve the safety of traditional circumcision practices. In South Africa, for example, laws have been passed by provincial governments in three provinces (e.g., the Application of Health Standards in Traditional Circumcision Act in the Eastern Cape Province) that aim to set safety standards for traditional health practitioners who carry out circumcision for cultural reasons. Similarly, in 2006, South Africa's parliament included a section on male circumcision in its Children' Act, which prohibited circumcision of males under 16 except when:

> "performed for religious purposes in accordance with the practices of the religion concerned and in the manner prescribed; or
>
> performed for medical reasons on the recommendation of a medical practitioner."

For children over 16 the law requires informed consent, proper counseling, and in "the manner prescribed."

References

Fenton, K. A. & T. A. Peterman, *HIV Partner Notification: Taking a New Look,* 11 *AIDS* 1535–46 (1997).

American Academy of Paediatrics Task Force on Circumcision, *Circumcision Policy Statement* 103 *Paediatrics* 666–93 (1999). http://aappolicy.aappublications.org/cgi/content/full/pediatrics%3b103/3/686

British Medical Association Committee on Medical Ethics, *The Law and Ethics of Male Circumcision—Guidance for Doctors* (June 2006). http://www.bma.org.uk/ap.nsf/Content/malecircumcision2006

Government of South Africa, *Application of Health Standards in Traditional Circumcision Act (Eastern Cape Province)* (2001). http://www.ecdoh.gov.za/policies_and_legislation/55/Application_of_Health_Standards_in_Traditional_Circumcision_Act

Republic of South Africa, Children's Act, No 38 of 2005. http://www.polity.org.za

UNAIDS, *Safe Male Circumcision and Comprehensive HIV Programming: Guidance for Decision Makers on Human Rights, Ethical and Legal Considerations* (2006).

WHO & UNAIDS, *New Data on Male Circumcision and HIV Prevention: Policy and Programme Implications* (March 2007). http://data.unaids.org/pub/Report/2007/mc_recomendations_en.pdf

WHO, UNAIDS, UNFPA, UNICEF, *World Bank Statement on Kenyan and Ugandan Trial Findings Regarding Male Circumcision and HIV* (December 2006). http://data.unaids.org/pub/PressStatement/2006/20061213_male_circumcision_joint_pr_en.pdf?preview=true

WHO & UNAIDS, *New Data on Male Circumcision and HIV Prevention: Policy and Programme Implications* (WHO/UNAIDS Technical Consultation on Male Circumcision and HIV Prevention: Research Implications for Policy and Programming Montreux, 6–8 March 2007, Conclusions and Recommendations). http://data.unaids.org/pub/Report/2007/mc_recommendations_en.pdf

Wilson, David & Joy de Beyer, *Male Circumcision: Evidence and Implications,* Getting Results, World Bank, Global HIV/AIDS Program (March 2006). http://www.worldbank.org/aids > Getting Results

SECTION 2

People Living with HIV: Discrimination

2.1 Protection Against Discrimination Based on HIV Status or Health Status

The Issue

Discrimination against persons living with HIV (PLHIV), as defined by the UNAIDS *Protocol for the Identification of Discrimination against People Living with HIV,* refers to "[a]ny measure entailing an arbitrary distinction among persons depending on their confirmed or suspected HIV serostatus or state of health." Discrimination against PLHIV may lead to intolerance and exacerbate the stigma PLHIV face regularly. Discrimination based on an infectious disease is just as inequitable as discrimination based on race, gender, or disability. HIV-positive persons do not present a health threat, and discrimination based on HIV or health status may compound the marginalization of groups already faced with stigma and societal opprobrium—groups like gay men, injecting drug users, and sex workers. Discrimination also undermines public health efforts to identify persons HIV-positive for the purposes of prevention of transmission, and provision of care and treatment. If individuals fear the personal, social, and economic consequences of being diagnosed with HIV or AIDS, they may forego testing, fail to discuss their health and risk behaviors with counselors, health care professionals, and their partners, and refrain from entering the health care system for treatment. Finally, by placing the focus of HIV infection on specific groups in the community, discrimination may breed complacency in other groups who wrongly assume that they are not at risk of HIV infection. Alleviating discrimination is consistent with efforts to respect, protect, and fulfill human rights and to prevent HIV and AIDS through public health initiatives.

Legal and Policy Considerations

Laws and policies that protect against discrimination based upon HIV status or health status more generally have been widely enacted. According to the *UNAIDS 2006 Report on the Global AIDS Epidemic,* 61% of countries report having laws or regulations that protect PLHIV from discrimination. These laws are embodied in antidiscrimination provisions found in international conventions and agreements, national constitutions and laws, and multiple court decisions affirming that arbitrary discrimination is wrong and damaging to society. Some laws and policies include "health status" or "disability" in the list of categories subject to protection from discrimination. Implementing regulations, policy guidance, and court interpretations have commonly found these terms to be broad enough to encompass HIV status, AIDS, or opportunistic infections and other health conditions related to HIV. Some laws additionally list HIV or AIDS as a specific category receiving protection against discrimination. Still others establish discrimination protections within HIV-specific or disability laws (see Topic 2.2).

The UNAIDS and OHCHR *International Guidelines* on *HIV/AIDS and Human Rights* set out several important features of antidiscrimination laws: 1) they should broadly apply to multiple areas, including health care, social security, welfare benefits, employment, education, sport, accommodations, clubs, trades unions, qualifying bodies, access to transport, and other services; 2) direct and indirect discrimination should be covered; and 3) redress should be available through independent, speedy, and effective legal procedures.

The inclusion of "health status" or "disability" as a protected category under antidiscrimination laws may have several advantages for PLHIV. First, using these general terms provides sufficient flexibility to grant protection from discrimination based upon HIV infection itself and a range of health conditions related to HIV (although there is no guarantee that general antidiscrimination provisions will be interpreted this broadly). The most comprehensive laws and policies extend protection to actual, perceived, or suspected HIV status to cover those who are discriminated against due to actual HIV-infection or the perception that they are infected because of proximity to others perceived to be infected (e.g., family members) or association with groups stereotypically linked with HIV infection. Second, the inclusion of health status in general antidiscrimination legislation typically provides protection against discrimination across multiple sectors in society. These laws often specifically apply antidiscrimination protections in major areas such as education, the workplace, health care, immigration, prisons, housing, insurance and benefits, access to credit, and civil rights generally (including rights to vote, marry, hold elected office, etc.). Third, coverage of health status in general antidiscrimination statutes ensures that HIV is treated like other health conditions. Finally, general antidiscrimination laws garner broader public support from multiple health constituencies than laws targeted at a single health condition like HIV.

Practice Examples

The Philippines *AIDS Control and Prevention Act of 1998* provides in Section 2 (Declaration of Policies) that ". . . discrimination, in all its forms and subtleties, against individuals with HIV or persons perceived or suspected of having HIV shall be considered inimical to individual and national interest . . ." and then establishes a number of specific prohibitions against discrimination in the workplace (Sec. 35), in schools (Sec. 36), in travel and habitation (Sec. 37), in public service (Sec. 38), in credit and insurance services (Sec. 39), in hospitals and health institutions (Sec. 40), and in burial services (Sec. 41), and provides penalties for "[a]ll discriminatory acts and policies referred to in this Act" (Sec. 42). (http://hivaidsclearinghouse.unesco.org/ev_en.php?ID=2050_201&ID2=DO_TOPIC)

The Bahamas has explicitly protected HIV and AIDS under the *Employment Act of 2001.* "No employer or person acting on behalf of an employer shall discriminate against an employee or applicant for employment on the basis of race, creed, sex, marital status, political opinion, age or HIV/AIDS." (Bahamas *Employment Act of 2001,* No. 73 of 2000, Sec. 6. http://www.lexbahamas.com/ Employment%20Act%202001.pdf)

South Africa's *Promotion of Equality and Prevention Unfair Discrimination Act No 4 of 2000* prohibits unfair discrimination in all sectors of society. The Act lists HIV as a directive principle on which discrimination cannot be grounded. (*Promotion of Equality and Prevention Unfair Discrimination Act No 4 of 2000,* South Africa, Schedule 5(c). http://www.polity.org.za/html/govdocs/legislation/ 2000/act4.pdf)

In New South Wales, Australia, the *Anti-Discrimination Act* makes it unlawful for a person "to incite hatred towards, serious contempt for, or severe ridicule of" anyone infected with HIV or thought to be HIV-positive. Under the law, serious HIV-related offenses include threatening physical harm or inciting others to threaten physical harm towards individuals or groups directly or to their property. (New South Wales Consolidated Act 48 of 1977. *Anti-Discrimination Act 1977.* http://www.austlii.edu.au/au/legis/nsw/consol_act/aa1977204/)

References

AIDS Law Project & AIDS Legal Network, *HIV/AIDS and the Law: A Resource Manual,* Chapter 2 (3rd ed., AIDS Law Project & AIDS Legal Network 2003).

Lawyers Collective, *Legislating an Epidemic: HIV/AIDS in India,* Chapter 1 (Universal Law Publishing Co. Pvt. Ltd. 2003).

National Aids Trust, *HIV-Related Stigma and Discrimination: Proposals from the National AIDS Trust for the Government Action Plan.* (National Aids Trust 2006) http://www.nat .org.uk/document/128

UNAIDS, *UNAIDS 2006 Report on the Global AIDS Epidemic* (UNAIDS 2006). http://www.unaids.org/en/HIV_data/2006GlobalReport/default.asp

————, *Protocol for the Identification of Discrimination against People Living with HIV* (UNAIDS 2000). http://data.unaids.org/Publications/IRC-pub01/JC295-Protocol_en.pdf

UNAIDS & OHCHR, *International Guidelines on HIV/AIDS and Human Rights,* 2006 Consolidated version (UNAIDS & Office of the United Nations High Commissioner for Human Rights 2006). http://data.unaids.org/Publications/IRC-pub07/JC1252-InternGuidelines_en.pdf?preview=true

United Nations Committee on Economic, Social, and Cultural Rights, *General Comment No. 14: The Right to the Highest Attainable Standard of Health* (Office of the United Nations High Commissioner for Human Rights 2000). http://www.unhchr.ch

United Nations Committee on the Rights of the Child, *General Comment No. 3: HIV/AIDS and the Rights of the Child* (Office of the United Nations High Commissioner for Human Rights 2003). http://www.unhchr.ch

2.2 Antidiscrimination Protection under Disability Laws

The Issue

Disability laws often define disability to include most serious medical conditions ranging from communicable diseases (TB, hepatitis, or syphilis) to chronic illnesses (like cerebral palsy, diabetes, or schizophrenia) that may result in a physical or mental impairment that substantially limits activity. In the United States and other countries disability has been defined or interpreted to include HIV-positive status, even when the infected person is asymptomatic.

Legal and Policy Considerations

Disability laws provide another framework within which PLHIV may receive legal protections against discrimination. Disability laws and HIV-specific laws differ from general discrimination laws in focus and form. In the realm of disability law, the focus is on providing opportunities and perhaps even affirmative services to persons with disabilities. Disability legislation commonly incorporates protections against discrimination based on disability into the legal framework to enhance the rights and social acceptance of persons with disabilities. Similarly, laws and policies enacted that are specific to HIV and AIDS often contain antidiscrimination provisions that bolster the public health and privacy initiatives found elsewhere in legislation or policy. By contrast, antidiscrimination laws tend to focus almost exclusively on protections against discrimination and categorize protected classes based upon factors such as race, gender, religion, or indeed, health status and disability (see Topic 2.1). PLHIV may benefit from legal protections against discrimination arising from both types of laws, and a number of countries have implemented both approaches simultaneously.

Some jurisdictions that have enacted disability laws—such as the United States, United Kingdom, and Hong Kong (China)—have based the applicability of discrimination protections on proof that the disability affects a person's ability to perform life functions, including work, education, and reproduction. Many countries have explicitly defined HIV as a disability under the law, or alternatively, courts have interpreted disability to include HIV and AIDS. Since discrimination is largely based on perception, many disability laws apply to persons perceived to have a disability as well as those whose functioning is actually affected by the disability. In some countries, designation of HIV as a disability also may entitle affected persons to health or other benefits. Much the same can be said about HIV-specific laws that provide antidiscrimination protections. Although these laws are less common than disability legislation, they are usually much clearer in their protection of actual or perceived HIV status.

One potential drawback to the disability law approach is that the scope of disability covered under law may fluctuate according to judicial interpretations, as has been the case with the *Americans with Disabilities Act* (ADA) in the United States. The ADA does not mention HIV or AIDS, or any other disabling conditions directly; instead, the statute describes the law's concept of a disability in general terms. Regulations and interpretative guidelines and early judicial decisions concerning the ADA solidified that HIV and AIDS both qualify as disabilities. However, the judiciary has more recently narrowed the scope of anti-discrimination protections granted to asymptomatic persons with HIV outside the work setting.

Practice Examples

In the United States, the *Americans with Disabilities Act* (ADA) proscribes discrimination against persons with disabilities in employment, public services, public accommodations, and telecommunications. A "person with a disability" is defined as someone who: (1) has a physical or mental impairment that substantially limits that person in one or more major life activities, or (2) has a record of such a physical or mental impairment, or (3) is regarded as having such a physical or mental impairment (United States 1990).

In the UK, the *Disability Discrimination Act* (DDA) of 2005 extended discrimination protections for those living with HIV to the moment of diagnosis. Previously, protection from discrimination began only from the moment someone with HIV became unable to carry out day-to-day tasks. Under the Act, discrimination is prohibited in the workplace, education, housing, trade union membership, and the provision of goods and services, including the buying and selling of property. Chapter 13, sec. 18 of the Act clearly includes HIV as a category of disability protected from discrimination: "a person who has cancer, HIV infection or multiple sclerosis is to be deemed to have a disability, and hence to be a disabled person" (United Kingdom 2005).

References

Supreme Court of the United States, *Bragdon v. Abbott, 524 U.S. 624. 1998*. (Cornell Law School Supreme Court Collection 1998) http://www.law.cornell.edu/supct/html/97-156.ZO.html

UNAIDS, *Protocol for the Identification of Discrimination against People Living with HIV* (UNAIDS 2000). http://data.unaids.org/Publications/IRC-pub01/JC295-Protocol_en.pdf

———, *UNAIDS 2006 Report on the Global AIDS Epidemic* (UNAIDS 2006). http://www.unaids.org/en/HIV_data/2006GlobalReport/default.asp

United Kingdom National AIDS Trust, *HIV-Related Stigma and Discrimination: Proposals from the National AIDS Trust for the Government Action Plan.* (National AIDS Trust 2006) http://www.nat.org.uk/document/128

United Kingdom Office of Public Sector Information, *Disability Discrimination Act of 2005* (OPSI 2005) http://www.opsi.gov.uk/acts/acts2005/20050013.htm

United States Department of Labor, *Americans with Disabilities Act or 1990, 42 U.S.C. § 12101 et seq* (Department of Labor April 12, 2007) http://www.dol.gov/esa/regs/statutes/ofccp/ada.htm

2.3 The Workplace: Testing at Recruitment and Mandatory Testing During Employment

The Issue

Discrimination in the workplace may present a substantial obstacle to persons living with HIV securing and maintaining employment. Despite laws in many countries prohibiting the use of HIV testing to discriminate against persons living with HIV, discrimination based upon HIV status continues to occur in the workplace. Some employers harbor misconceptions about the routes of HIV transmission and fear increased HIV transmission within their workplace, while others fear increased costs, including health care and insurance costs and expenses to accommodate employees living with HIV. Most persons living with HIV can work normally or with minimal accommodations. Yet, many employers insist on using HIV testing requirements to screen potential employees during the hiring process and to eliminate HIV-infected employees from their workforce.

Legal and Policy Considerations

Laws and policies in many countries restrict employers from testing potential or current employees for HIV. These laws and policies take several forms—some proscribe mandatory HIV testing during recruiting, employment, or both. One common approach adopted in many laws prohibits mandatory HIV testing from the beginning of the hiring process throughout the employee's tenure at the workplace. With these protections in place, employees cannot be compelled to undergo HIV testing at any time without their consent. Moreover, test results or the failure to undergo testing cannot be used as a basis for denying employment, promotion, training, or benefits to an employee. The *ILO Code of Practice on HIV/AIDS and the World of Work* supports this position, stating: "HIV testing should not be required at the time of recruitment or as a condition of continued employment." Another approach provides even more privacy protection: forbidding HIV testing of applicants during recruiting even with their informed consent. This strong prohibition on HIV testing during recruitment recognizes that informed consent given by prospective employees may, in fact, have elements of coercion. Most laws that address workplace testing permit HIV testing with informed consent.

Laws and policies that prohibit mandatory HIV testing in the workplace setting place a high value on protecting the privacy of job applicants and current employees, and seek to avoid discrimination and stigma in the workplace. Mandatory HIV testing has no practical application in the workplace because employee evaluations must be based upon the employee's job performance, not his or her diagnosis. Test results, even if not misused in workplace decision-making (e.g., assignments, promotion, and training opportunities), may become known to others in the workplace, resulting in embarrassment and marginalization for an employee. Laws proscribing mandatory testing also frequently prohibit HIV status from being considered as a factor that will affect continued employment (see Topic 2.4) or result in differential treatment (see Topic 2.5). Furthermore, legal protections also may extend to protection of benefits. Mandatory testing for HIV should not be required to qualify for life and health insurance, pensions, and other benefits afforded to employees (see Topic 2.11).

Many laws, however, do permit HIV testing of staff in health care settings due to the increased chance of HIV exposure through contact with bodily fluids. Hospitals in many countries implement the use of universal precautions so that infected hospital workers pose minimal risk to patients (and to reduce the risk of infection for workers). Amid controversy, some countries have authorized testing of employees engaged in seriously invasive procedures to address concerns about the risk infected workers may pose to patients.

Enforceability of laws prohibiting mandatory HIV testing in the workplace provides another challenge. For example, even in countries that prohibit HIV testing of employees, employers may ask employees to be tested, and dismiss employees who test positive for HIV.

Practice Examples

In Zimbabwe, the *Labour Relations (HIV and AIDS) Regulations* prohibit mandatory HIV testing during recruitment and for employees. "No employer shall require, whether directly or indirectly, any person to undergo any form of testing for HIV as a precondition to the offer of employment . . . It shall not be compulsory for any employee to undergo, directly or indirectly, any testing for HIV." (http://www.ilo.org/public/english/protection/trav/aids/laws/zimbabweregs.pdf)

In Malawi, the *Malawi National HIV/AIDS Policy* guarantees all people freedom from discrimination on the grounds of HIV or AIDS status. Concerning the workplace, the policy prohibits employers from requiring any person to undergo testing for HIV as a precondition for employment. The policy stresses that the criteria for employment must be fitness and ability to do the job. (http://www.ilo.org/public/english/protection/trav/aids/laws/malawinationalpolicy.pdf)

The Bahamas protect persons living with HIV from workplace HIV testing under Section 6(c) of the *Employment Act of 2001*. "No employer or person acting on behalf of an employer shall discriminate against an employee or applicant for employment on the basis of . . . HIV/AIDS . . . by pre-screening for HIV status" (Government of Bahamas 2001).

South Africa's Employment Equity Act (No. 55 of 1998), Sec. 7(2) specifically prohibits HIV testing of employees "unless such testing is determined justifiable by the Labour Court in terms of section 50(4) of this Act." Section 50(4) provides that if upon application of an employer the Labour Court declares that such medical testing is justifiable, the Labour Court's order may include "imposing conditions relating to: (a) the provision of counseling; (b) the maintenance of confidentiality; (c) the period during which the authorization for any testing applies; and (d) the category or categories of jobs or employees in respect of which the authorization for testing applies." (http://www.labour.gov.za/act/index. jsp?legislationId=59548actID=8191)

References

Government of Bahamas, *Employment Act of 2001,* No. 73 of 2000, Sec. 6 (Government of Bahamas 2000). http://www.lexbahamas.com/Employment%20Act%202001.pdf

ILO, *An ILO Code of Practice on HIV/AIDS and the World of Work,* Sec. 8 (International Labour Organization 2001). http://www.ilo.org/public/english/protection/trav/aids/publ/code.htm

————, *Implementing the ILO Code of Practice on HIV/AIDS and the World of Work: An Education and Training Manual,* Module 2 (International Labour Organization 2002). http://www.ilo.org/public/english/protection/trav/aids/publ/manual.htm

ILO & UNESCO, *Workplace Policies on HIV and AIDS for the Education Sector: Joint ILO/UNESCO Programme* (United Nations Educational, Scientific, and Cultural Organization 2006). http://portal.unesco.org/fr/ev.php-URL_ID=34833&URL_DO=DO_TOPIC&URL_SECTION=201.html

SADC, *National and Sector HIV/AIDS Policies in the Member States of the Southern Africa Development Community* (Southern African Development Community 2002).

Rwebangira, M. K. & M. B. Tungaraza, *Review and Assessment of Laws Affecting HIV/AIDS in Tanzania,* Nov., Chapter 9 (Tanzania Women Lawyers' Association 2003). http://www.policyproject.com/pubs/countryreports/TZlawreview_sumbooklet.pdf http://www.policyproject.com/pubs/countryreports/TZlawreview.pdf (Full report)

UNAIDS, *A Human Rights Approach to AIDS Prevention at Work: The Southern African Development Community's Code on HIV/AIDS and Employment,* UNAIDS Best Practice Collection, June (UNAIDS 2000). http://www.unaids.org

2.4 The Workplace: Denial of Employment

The Issue

Discrimination in the workplace may occur when a person is denied employment because of his or her actual or perceived HIV status. Discrimination resulting in a denial of employment can arise during the hiring and recruitment process or when an existing employee is terminated as a consequence of his or her HIV status. In addition to denial of employment, HIV status might also be used to limit an employee's opportunities, such as for a promotion. Many laws prevent employers from compelling HIV testing (see Topic 2.3) or disclosure of HIV status (see Topic 2.6) of a prospective or current employee. However, an employee's HIV status may become known to the employer through a variety of circumstances, including voluntary disclosure by the employee, medical and insurance reports sent to the employer (although these may be protected by privacy laws), or through a third party revealing this information to the employer. Once the employer is privy to an employee's HIV-positive status, some employers will attempt to terminate the employee based on this information. Consequently, many countries have enacted laws that protect HIV-positive persons in recruitment, hiring, and employment.

Legal and Policy Considerations

Denial of employment based upon HIV status violates antidiscrimination laws and policies in many countries. Labor and employment legislation and policies often provide generalized protection from discrimination that results in a denial of employment. These laws may specifically prohibit an employer from refusing to hire an applicant or from firing an employee based upon HIV status. More often, courts have defined the antidiscrimination provisions in labor and employment legislation to apply in the context of HIV status. In some countries, courts also have interpreted general antidiscrimination provisions in legislation or constitutional provisions to prohibit denial of employment based upon HIV status.

In countries with strong antidiscrimination laws protecting HIV-positive persons from denial of employment, employers do not have the right to know the HIV status of an applicant or employee and should not attempt to discover this information. To satisfy the antidiscrimination requirements, employers must strive to create employment security for workers living with HIV until they can no longer work. This may include providing them with certain reasonable accommodations such as flexibility in working hours to schedule doctor's appointments, flexible sick leave, special equipment, access to quiet areas for breaks, and access to kitchen facilities for preparation of food required by their therapy. The *ILO Code of Practice for HIV/AIDS and the World of Work* summarizes this point effectively: "HIV infection is not a cause for termination of employment. As with many other conditions, persons with HIV-related illnesses should be encouraged to work for as long as medically fit in available, appropriate work."

Despite increasing recognition of antidiscrimination protection for HIV-positive employees, discrimination and denial of employment continue to occur. Limits on enforceability of antidiscrimination laws related to HIV status in the workplace remain a major hindrance in protecting people with HIV.

Practice Examples

The Bahamas has explicitly protected PLHIV from denial of employment based on HIV status under section 6(a) of the *Employment Act of 2001.* "No employer or person acting on behalf of an employer shall discriminate against an employee or applicant for employment on the basis of . . . HIV/AIDS . . . by refusing to offer employment to an applicant for employment or . . . by dismissing or subjecting the employee to other detriment solely because of . . . HIV/AIDS." (http://www .lexbahamas.com/Employment%20Act%202001.pdf)

In a 1997 decision, the Bombay High Court in India ordered public sector companies to employ HIV-positive workers. The Court held that a company could not deny employment to an HIV-positive person "merely on the ground of his HIV status irrespective of his ability to perform the job requirements and irrespective of the fact that he does not pose any threat to others at the workplace" finding these actions to be "clearly arbitrary and unreasonable" under the Constitution of India. (*MX v. ZY,* AIR 1997 Bom 406 High Court of Judicature)

The Philippines *AIDS Prevention and Control Act 1998,* Section 35 generally prohibits discrimination in the workplace and provides clear employment protection for HIV-positive workers, stating that "[t]ermination of work on the sole basis of actual, perceived or suspected HIV status is deemed unlawful." (http://hivaidsclearinghouse.unesco.org/ev_en.php?ID=2050_201&ID2=DO_ TOPIC)

In Zimbabwe, the *Labour Relations (HIV and AIDS) Regulations* state that "[n]o employer shall terminate the employment of an employee on the grounds of that employee's HIV status alone." (http://www.ilo.org/public/ english/protection/trav/aids/laws/zimbabweregs.pdf)

In *Hoffmann v. South African Airways* the Constitutional Court of South Africa ruled that the national airline's policy of refusing to hire HIV positive people violated the country's constitutional protection of equal rights. UNAIDS/Canadian HIV/AIDS Legal Network. Courting Rights: Case Studies in Litigating the Human Rights of People Living with HIV. (http://www.aidslaw.ca/publications/ publicationsdocEN.php?ref=45)

References

AIDS Law Project & AIDS Legal Network, *HIV/AIDS and the Law: A Resource Manual,* Chapter 7 (3rd ed., AIDS Law Project & AIDS Legal Network 2003).

ILO, *An ILO Code of Practice on HIV/AIDS and the World of Work,* sec. 8 (International Labour Organization 2001). http://www.ilo.org/public/english/protection/trav/aids/publ/code.htm

———, *Implementing the ILO Code of Practice on HIV/AIDS and the World of Work: An Education and Training Manual,* Module 2 (International Labour Organization 2002). http://www.ilo.org/public/english/protection/trav/aids/publ/manual.htm

ILO & UNESCO, *Workplace Policies on HIV and AIDS for the Education Sector: Joint ILO/UNESCO Programme* (United Nations Educational, Scientific, and Cultural Organization 2006) http://portal.unesco.org/fr/ev.php-URL_ID=34833&URL_DO=DO_TOPIC &URL_SECTION=201.html

Lawyers' Collective, *Legislating an Epidemic: HIV/AIDS in India,* Chapter 1 (Universal Law Publishing Co. Pvt. Ltd. 2003).

Rwebangira, M. K. & M. B. Tungaraza, *Review and Assessment of Laws Affecting HIV/AIDS in Tanzania,* Nov., Chapter 9 (Tanzania Women Lawyers' Association 2003). http://www.policyproject.com/pubs/countryreports/TZlawreview_sumbooklet.pdf http://www.policyproject.com/pubs/countryreports/TZlawreview.pdf (Full report)

SADC, *National and Sector HIV/AIDS Policies in the Member States of the Southern Africa Development Community* (Southern African Development Community 2002).

UNAIDS, *A Human Rights Approach to AIDS Prevention at Work: The Southern African Development Community's Code on HIV/AIDS and Employment,* UNAIDS Best Practice Collection, June (UNAIDS 2000). http://www.unaids.org

2.5   The Workplace: Differential Treatment

The Issue

Employees living with HIV are often subjected to differential treatment in the workplace by their employers, coworkers, unions, or clients. Employers discriminate against HIV-positive employees by providing them less opportunities within the workplace—for increased wages, promotions, assignments, insurance, pensions, health benefits, etc.—compared with other employees. Differential treatment prevails within the workplace because employers, coworkers, and others may misunderstand and fear an HIV-positive employee and ostracize him or her as contagious or immoral. Employers may have a misperception that HIV-positive employees are less productive than other employees, and colleagues may marginalize HIV-positive employees through threats, ridicule, and malicious gossip. Employers who do not protect HIV-positive employees from stigmatization by colleagues, clients, and others engage in discrimination by allowing this adverse treatment to continue. Along with other forms of workplace discrimination, such as refusing to hire applicants who are HIV-positive or firing employees due to their HIV status (see Topics 2.3, 2.4), differential treatment discriminates against employees with HIV because they are not afforded the same treatment, consideration, and respect as other employees.

In addition, employers may discriminate against HIV-positive employees by not providing them with certain types of beneficial treatment based on their needs. In order to facilitate the workplace performance of HIV-positive employees, an employer may need to provide reasonable accommodations for their health needs.

Legal and Policy Considerations

Laws that protect the rights of employees living with HIV exist in many countries, and these laws frequently include provisions protecting employees from differential treatment in the workplace based upon their HIV status. These protections may be stated generally (HIV status may not be used as a justification to treat workers differently than similarly situated workers) or may apply specifically to particular areas of.the workplace setting (e.g., to fairness in promotions or access to benefits). In countries without specific workplace antidiscrimination laws, general antidiscrimination provisions may prevent differential treatment based upon HIV status. Even in the absence of legal requirements or government directives, some employers have on their own initiative prohibited discrimination against employees based on HIV status.

Legal frameworks may provide HIV-positive workers with protections against differential treatment, but laws have not always changed people's mindsets. The best way to prevent differential treatment in the workplace is to keep the HIV status of employees confidential (see Topic 2.6). However, if other employees or customers do discover the HIV status of an employee, education efforts are vital to prevent discrimination against HIV-positive employees. The ILO recommends that workplaces develop education and training in the workplace related to HIV and AIDS to reduce discrimination and differential treatment. If employers, coworkers, and customers understand the nature of HIV infection and that HIV cannot be transmitted through casual contact, differential treatment in the workplace will be less likely to occur.

In countries where HIV infection qualifies as a disability, HIV-positive employees may have the right to reasonable adjustments if any practices and premises place them at a substantial disadvantage. For example, an employer may have to adjust the employee's schedule to accommodate the employee's leave time for treatment. This type of differential treatment is necessary, and often required, to accommodate the needs of HIV-positive employees. The OHCHR and WHO support employment security for HIV-positive workers that may be aided by reasonable alternative working arrangements.

Practice Examples

In South Africa, the *Employment Equity Act of 1998* states, "no person may unfairly discriminate, directly or indirectly, against an employee, in any employment policy or practice, on one or more grounds, including . . . HIV status." (http://www.scienceinafrica.co.za/2002/december/hivwork.htm)

In Zimbabwe, the *Labour Relations (HIV and AIDS) Regulations* prohibit differential treatment in the workplace based on HIV status. "No employee shall be prejudiced in relation to (a) promotion; or (b) transfer; or (c) subject to any other law to the contrary, any training or other employee development programme; or (d) status; or in any other way, be discriminated against on the grounds of his HIV status alone." (http://www.ilo.org/public/english/protection/trav/aids/laws/zimbabweregs.pdf)

Section 6(a) of the Bahamas *Employment Act of 2001* provides that "[n]o employer or person acting on behalf of an employer shall discriminate against an employee or applicant for employment on the basis of . . . HIV/AIDS . . . by not affording the employee access to opportunities for promotion, training or other benefits." (http://www.lexbahamas.com/Employment%20Act%202001.pdf)

References

AIDS Law Project & AIDS Legal Network, *HIV/AIDS and the Law: A Resource Manual*, Chapter 7 (3rd ed., AIDS Law Project & AIDS Legal Network 2003). http://www.alp.org.za

ILO, *An ILO Code of Practice on HIV/AIDS and the World of Work,* Secs. 4,6,7,9 (International Labour Organization 2001). http://www.ilo.org/public/english/protection/trav/aids/publ/ code.htm

————, *Implementing the ILO Code of Practice on HIV/AIDS and the World of Work: An Education and Training Manual,* Module 2 (International Labour Organization 2002). http:// www.ilo.org/public/english/protection/trav/aids/publ/manual.htm

ILO & UNESCO, *Workplace Policies on HIV and AIDS for the Education Sector: Joint ILO/UNESCO Programme* (United Nations Educational, Scientific, and Cultural Organization 2006). http://portal.unesco.org/fr/ev.php-URL_ID=34833&URL_DO=DO_TOPIC &URL_SECTION=201.html

Lawyers' Collective, *Legislating an Epidemic: HIV/AIDS in India,* Chapter 1 (Universal Law Publishing Co. Pvt. Ltd. 2003).

SADC, *National and Sector HIV/AIDS Policies in the Member States of the Southern Africa Development Community* (Southern African Development Community 2002).

UNAIDS, *A Human Rights Approach to AIDS Prevention at Work: The Southern African Development Community's Code on HIV/AIDS and Employment,* UNAIDS Best Practice Collection, June (UNAIDS 2000). http://www.unaids.org

United Kingdom National AIDS Trust, *HIV @ Work Pack* (National AIDS Trust 2006). http://www.nat.org.uk/document/129

2.6 The Workplace: Disclosure and Confidentiality

The Issue

Discrimination in the workplace may occur when information about an employee's HIV status is revealed to an employer, coworkers, or clients. Employees who are living with HIV often have a strong incentive to keep their HIV status confidential to avoid negative or unfair treatment by their employers and stigmatization by their coworkers. Efforts to compel disclosure of HIV status violate the employee's privacy and autonomy. Furthermore, except in rare circumstances, HIV infection cannot be transmitted through normal workplace interaction, and thus poses no immediate safety risk in the workplace. Laws and policies prohibiting disclosure of HIV status without consent and otherwise limiting access to HIV information can protect HIV-positive persons from potential discrimination in the workplace.

Legal and Policy Considerations

Several types of laws protect the confidentiality of HIV-related information in the workplace. In countries that have enacted generally applicable confidentiality protections for HIV information or medical records, these protections may extend to disclosure of HIV information in the workplace. However, general privacy and confidentiality laws may only apply to HIV information in certain settings (e.g., health care), so it may be necessary to enact HIV confidentiality laws that apply directly to the workplace. These provisions may directly apply confidentiality protections for HIV information in the possession of employers or, alternatively, they may protect employee confidentiality by preventing employers from requiring HIV testing or disclosure by employees of their HIV status. The *ILO Code of Practice on HIV/AIDS and the World of Work* takes a strong position for confidentiality protections and against compelled disclosure. "There is no justification for asking job applicants or workers to disclose HIV-related personal information. Nor should co-workers be obliged to reveal such personal information about fellow workers. Access to personal data relating to a worker's HIV status should be bound by the rules of confidentiality."

Privacy laws with confidentiality provisions that extend to employers may protect medical and insurance reports sent to the employer. Laws and policies also may limit access to HIV information to only those who need to know the information for administering benefits. The *ILO Code of Practice* endorses this approach as well. "Governments, private insurance companies and employers should ensure that information relating to counselling, care, treatment and receipt of benefits is kept confidential . . . Third parties, such as trustees and administrators of social security programmes and occupational schemes, should keep all HIV/AIDS-related information confidential, as with medical data pertinent to workers."

Practice Examples

Zimbabwe's *Labour Relations (HIV/AIDS) Regulations of 1998* provide disclosure and confidentiality protections in the workplace: "No employer shall require any employee, and it shall not be compulsory for any employee, to disclose, in respect of any matter whatsoever in connection with his employment, his HIV status . . . No person shall, except with the written consent of the employee to whom the information relates, disclose any information relating to the HIV status of any employee acquired by that person in the course of his duties unless the information is required to be disclosed in terms of any other law." (http://www.ilo.org/public/english/protection/trav/aids/laws/zimbabweregs.pdf)

In Cambodia, the *Law of Prevention and Control of HIV/AIDS* requires that the confidentiality of all persons living with HIV is maintained by "health professionals, workers, employers, recruitment agencies, insurance companies, data encoders, custodians of medical records related to HIV/AIDS, and those who have the relevant duties" shall maintain the confidentiality, including the identity and personal status, of persons living with HIV. (http://www.ilo.org/public/english/protection/trav/aids/laws/cambodia1.pdf)

The *Malawi National HIV/AIDS Policy* states: "No employee shall be compelled to disclose his or her HIV status to their employer or other employees. Where an employee chooses to voluntarily disclose his or her HIV status to the employer or to another employee, such information shall not be disclosed to others without that employee's express written consent." (http://www.ilo.org/public/english/protection/trav/aids/laws/malawinationalpolicy.pdf)

References

AIDS Law Project & AIDS Legal Network, *HIV/AIDS and the Law: A Resource Manual*, Chapter 7 (3rd ed., AIDS Law Project & AIDS Legal Network 2003).

ILO, *An ILO Code of Practice on HIV/AIDS and the World of Work*, Sec. 8 (International Labour Organization 2001). http://www.ilo.org/public/english/protection/trav/aids/publ/code.htm

———, *Implementing the ILO Code of Practice on HIV/AIDS and the World of Work: An Education and Training Manual*, Module 2 (International Labour Organization 2002). http://www.ilo.org/public/english/protection/trav/aids/publ/manual.htm

ILO & UNESCO, *Workplace Policies on HIV and AIDS for the Education Sector: Joint ILO/UNESCO Programme* (United Nations Educational, Scientific, and Cultural Organization 2006). http://portal.unesco.org/fr/ev.php-URL_ID=34833&URL_DO=DO_TOPIC&URL_SECTION=201.html

UNAIDS, *A Human Rights Approach to AIDS Prevention at Work: The Southern African Development Community's Code on HIV/AIDS and Employment,* UNAIDS Best Practice Collection, June (UNAIDS 2000). http://www.unaids.org

2.7   Health Care: Refusal to Treat

The Issue

Gaining access to health care is one of the most successful methods for controlling the HIV epidemic. However, around the world PLHIV and those perceived as being infected with HIV continue to face discrimination in the health care sector. Doctors, nurses, and other health professionals may harbor the same fears, ignorance, and aversions as other members of the population with regard to HIV. In the health care setting, these attitudes can lead to discrimination that prevents PLHIV from accessing health care.

Discrimination can manifest in outright refusals to admit or treat patients who are infected with HIV or perceived as infected, delays and withholding of care or treatment to these patients, and premature discharge of patients. These actions may have consequences beyond preventing access to treatment for HIV or AIDS; access to all health care services may be undermined. By refusing to treat patients, the risk of serious health consequences increases for both the individual and the general population. Lack of resources in the health care system also may provoke discrimination against PLHIV, when scarce resources are intentionally reserved for other patients.

Legal and Policy Considerations

Direct denials of care on the basis of HIV status are often prohibited under general antidiscrimination legislation or through disability or HIV-specific laws. Some countries have chosen to enact specific protections against discrimination based on HIV status in the health sector within national legislation or policy. Legal frameworks that address the workplace and occupational health and safety issues also may contribute to antidiscrimination protections.

While antidiscrimination laws and policies provide a clear message that it is inappropriate to refuse to treat HIV-positive persons due to their HIV status, the nature of many health care systems allows discrimination to continue under the guise of resource allocation decisions. Under the law in many countries, private hospitals and other health institutions are not required to accept all patients and may not be covered by antidiscrimination provisions (which may only apply to government or public sector health care institutions). Private health care institutions may refuse to provide nonemergency care to a patient who cannot pay. In this case, the courts may need to determine whether the refusal to treat a patient occurred due to the patient's HIV status—which would be prohibited under antidiscrimination laws—or because of other, legitimate justifications. In other countries, antidiscrimination laws apply to all health care institutions and settings (see Cambodia example below).

Some national HIV and AIDS policies emphasize training efforts to educate health care workers about the low risks of contracting HIV at work and to reduce stigma and the occurrence of discrimination in the health sector. The Pan American Health Organization has identified several factors that can reduce discriminatory attitudes among health workers: "(a) accurate knowledge of the means of transmission and nontransmission of HIV, (b) skill in interacting appropriately with patients with HIV/AIDS, (c) regular contact with people with the virus, (d) techniques to avoid burnout, and (e) awareness of human rights norms that protect patients with HIV/AIDS and of the consequences of violating those norms."

Practice Examples

In Cambodia, the *Law of Prevention and Control of HIV/AIDS* strictly prohibits the refusal of health care on the basis of HIV or AIDS status. Article 41 states, "No person shall be denied to receive public and private health care services or be charged with higher fee on the basis of the actual, perceived or suspected HIV/AIDS status of the person or his/her family members." (http://www. ilo.org/public/english/protection/trav/aids/laws/cambodia1.pdf)

In the Philippines, the *AIDS Prevention and Control Act 1998,* outlaws discrimination based upon HIV status in hospitals and health institutions. Under Section 40 of the Act, "No person shall be denied health care service or be charged with a higher fee on account of actual, perceived or suspected HIV status." (http://www.doh.gov.ph/pnacwebsite/RA8504.pdf)

References

Human Rights Watch, *Future Forsaken: Abuses Against Children Affected by HIV/AIDS in India* (Human Rights Watch 2004). http://hrw.org/reports/2004/india0704/FutureForsaken .pdf

ILO & WHO, *Joint ILO/WHO Guidelines on Health Services and HIV/AIDS* (International Labour Organization & World Health Organization 2005). www.ilo.org/public/english/ dialogue/sector/techmeet/tmehs05/guidelines.pdf

Lawyers' Collective, *Legislating an Epidemic: HIV/AIDS in India,* Chapter 12 (Universal Law Publishing Co. Pvt. Ltd. 2003).

Pan American Health Organization, *Understanding and Responding to HIV/AIDS-Related Stigma and Discrimination in the Health Sector* (Pan American Health Organization 2003). http://www.paho.org/English/AD/FCH/AI/stigma.htm

UNAIDS & WHO, *Fighting HIV-related intolerance: exposing the links between racism, stigma and discrimination,* prepared in consultation with the Office of the High Commissioner for Human Rights (UNAIDS & WHO c.2001). http://www.unhchr.ch/html/ menu2/7/b/hivbpracism.doc

UNAIDS, *Policy Brief: Antiretroviral Therapy and Injecting Drug Users* (UNAIDS 2005). http://www.wpro.who.int/NR/rdonlyres/539F9FB1-0801-49B9-BAFF-B6FF88EF6583/0/ antiretroviraltherapy.pdf

UNDP, *Law, Ethics and HIV/AIDS in South Asia: A Study of the Legal and Social Environment of the Epidemic in Bangladesh, India, Nepal and Sri Lanka* (United Nations Development Programme 2002). http://www.undprcc.lk/Publications/Publications/Law EthicsandHIVAIDS.pdf

2.8   Health Care: Differential Treatment

The Issue

Discrimination in the form of disparate health care treatment based upon HIV status has been reported in many countries. Fear of transmission and disapproval of the actual or presumed lifestyles of patients may fuel discrimination by health care workers. The list of discriminatory practices documented in the health sector is long and varied and includes: testing without consent, breaches of confidentiality, refusing to inform patients of HIV-positive test results, inappropriate comments or behavior, use of excessive precautions, physical isolation or restriction of movement, charging excessive fees, and restrictions on access to basic necessities such as eating utensils and toilet facilities. Some health care workers may feel that HIV-positive patients are to blame for their condition and treat them with less compassion than other patients. Differential treatment can lead to negative health outcomes for patients with HIV or AIDS because they may not receive the care they need. Finally, discrimination in the health sector undermines public health efforts to identify persons infected with HIV, prevent transmission, and provide humane care and effective treatment to all PLHIV.

Legal and Policy Considerations

Numerous countries have enacted and implemented prohibitions against discriminatory treatment on the basis of HIV status in health care settings. Protections against discrimination in the health care setting may arise from general antidiscrimination laws or from provisions that specifically proscribe differential treatment and other forms of discrimination in the health sector. Antidiscrimination protections may apply to institutional actors (e.g., hospitals, health institutions), to health care workers themselves, or both. HIV-specific legislation and regulations protecting confidentiality, requiring informed consent, and promoting training and education also help reduce discrimination by fostering equitable practices and a more informed understanding of HIV by those working in the health sector.

In countries where legislation specifically prohibits discrimination against HIV-positive patients in facilities where HIV patients are likely to be treated, HIV-positive individuals may still be subject to discrimination in other facilities that provide health care services but do not provide HIV care. Even though these other facilities provide services unrelated to HIV, they often discriminate against HIV-positive patients, treating them after other patients out of a misguided perception that they are "lost causes" anyway. Countries that have enacted broader antidiscrimination laws covering all areas of health care services may provide more consistent protections to prevent differential treatment of HIV-positive persons throughout the health care system.

Professional codes of conduct and other policy documents may bolster efforts to reduce discrimination in the health care setting. Ethical codes, often drafted by associations representing health professionals, may complement legal requirements and require health care professionals to adhere to consistent standards when treating HIV-positive patients. These codes and standards are limited in that they typically only apply to specific categories of professionals and therefore do not inform the actions of all workers in the health sector. Furthermore, they are not enforceable under law if violations occur. Both laws and ethical standards support the notion that all patients should be entitled to quality standards of practice from health care workers regardless of the specific health condition or disease that they have. If health care workers believe that a patient's condition poses a serious risk to their safety, they may take reasonable measures to protect themselves, but they may not alter the standard of the care that the patient receives. "Reasonable" is a relative term, so this standard can be controversial in its implementation. However, certain practices, such as the implementation of universal precautions in the health care setting (see Topic 1.9), reduce differential treatment of patients and thereby reduce discrimination against PLHIV.

Practice Examples

Article 41 of the Cambodia *Law on the Prevention and Control of HIV/AIDS* states "Discrimination against persons with HIV/AIDS in the hospitals and health institutions is strictly prohibited. No person shall be denied to receive public and private health care services or be charged with higher fee on the basis of the actual, perceived or suspected HIV/AIDS status of the person or his/her family members." (http://www.ilo.org/public/english/protection/trav/aids/laws/cambodia1.pdf)

The Guyana *National Policy on HIV/AIDS* emphasizes the rights of "[a]ll HIV positive individuals, regardless of nationality, race, age, religion, disabilities, gender, sexual orientation and socio-economic status . . . to the best quality of health care available without being subjected to any form of discrimination." Guyana's government has also promoted various programs, such as making free antiretroviral medication available to all people living with AIDS, training doctors on how to treat patients with HIV, and raising HIV awareness in remote rural communities. (http://www.hiv.gov.gy/docs/nac_po_revisedaidspolicy.pdf)

In South Africa, the Health Professions Council of South Africa has issued guidelines that impose ethical obligations on health care workers to not "withhold normal standards of treatment from any patient solely on the grounds that the patient is seropositive, unless such variation of treatment is determined to be in the patient's interest. Treatment should not be suboptimal because of a perceived potential risk to the health care workers. It is accepted that a health care worker will examine or treat a patient only with the informed consent of the patient." (http://alp.org.za/images/upload/3rdAids%20finalss%20append.pdf)

References

Aids Law Project & AIDS Legal Network, *HIV/AIDS and the Law: A Resource Manual,* Chapter 6: 146–48 (3rd ed., Aids Law Project & AIDS Legal Network 2003). http://www.alp.org.za/

Bulkan, Arif, *HIV/AIDS, Law, and Discrimination in Guyana,* HIV/AIDS Law and Policy Review (9) (Canadian HIV/AIDS Legal Network December 2004). http://www.aidslaw.ca/publications/publicationsdocEN.php?ref=258

ILO & WHO, *Joint ILO/WHO Guidelines on Health Services and HIV/AIDS* (International Labour Organization and World Health Organization 2005). www.ilo.org/public/english/dialogue/sector/techmeet/tmehs05/guidelines.pdf

Pan American Health Organization, *Understanding and Responding to HIV/AIDS-related Stigma and Discrimination in the Health Sector* (Pan American Health Organization 2003). http://www.paho.org/English/AD/FCH/AI/stigma.htm

UNAIDS, *Policy Brief: Antiretroviral Therapy and Injecting Drug Users* (UNAIDS 2005). http://www.wpro.who.int/NR/rdonlyres/539F9FB1-0801-49B9-BAFF-B6FF88EF6583/0/antiretroviraltherapy.pdf

2.9   Issues at the Border: Travel and Immigration Restrictions

The Issue

Many countries impose restrictions on HIV-positive persons entering into the country. These restrictions may apply to short-term visitors (travelers, for business or personal visits, or tourism) or long-term visitors (students, workers, refugees, immigrants). Protection of the public from communicable diseases is a traditional ground to deny would-be visitors or immigrants entrance to countries. These restrictions are designed to prevent the introduction of infectious diseases into susceptible populations and to prevent infected visitors or immigrants from becoming a public charge. Laws and policies that restrict entry based on HIV status or that require a declaration of HIV status or HIV testing are frequently criticized as being ineffective at stopping the spread of HIV and imposing undue and arbitrary restrictions on personal liberty.

Legal and Policy Considerations

In general, national governments have the legal authority and discretion to restrict entry into their country, so long as these restrictions do not contradict international treaties to which they are members or violate domestic laws pertaining to travel or immigration. A common approach used by many countries requires those seeking to enter the country to declare their HIV status or submit to an HIV test. Most countries that have adopted these approaches only target long-term stays—usually six months or more—or permanent residency for HIV-positive people. However, a few countries, including the United States, bar any person who declares that they are HIV-positive from entry to the country, usually with the opportunity to apply for a waiver.

Countries that have entry restrictions based on HIV status generally justify them on public health grounds. The argument is that by screening for and denying entry of persons with HIV, a country could prevent the introduction and propagation of the disease within the country. Additionally, because many people with HIV are asymptomatic, testing may provide early detection and the ability for people to seek treatment earlier in the course of the disease (although most countries with restrictive entry policies do not provide HIV counseling or treatment services to persons at the border). A second common justification used for HIV entry restrictions is that limiting entry of HIV-positive persons will reduce the cost of treatment and care for HIV and AIDS that long-term visitors or immigrants will incur within the health system.

Nevertheless, entry restrictions and requirements for HIV declaration and testing are particularly unhelpful from a public health standpoint. Unlike many other communicable diseases that may justify entry restrictions, HIV cannot be transmitted through casual contact. There is no evidence that entry restrictions have a significant effect on the prevention of HIV transmission. Most countries do not screen or exclude returning nationals for HIV. Testing may produce false positives or negatives and may not detect persons recently infected with HIV because they have not yet produced HIV antibodies. Further, it is relatively easy to get around declaration requirements, particularly if there is no testing to confirm the veracity of one's declarations. While long-term visitors and immigrants who are HIV positive may indeed require public health care services, and therefore add to the charges on the state's public health budget, such a financial argument to justify the entry exclusion would be discriminatory as there are no entry exclusions for people with other high-cost diseases such as, for example, cancer.

Practice Examples

Iceland has one of the most progressive and accommodating programs for travelers and immigrants with HIV. There are no travel restrictions for people with HIV, and neither a declaration nor a test is required. A health exam is required when one applies for a permit to become a permanent resident. However, if health authorities determine that someone has HIV during this process, they are not restricted from obtaining permanent resident status. Instead, they are immediately enrolled in the national health care service, and the usual six month residency requirement for entry into the health service is waived (Aidsnet 2003).

Cambodia does not restrict residency or travel on the basis of HIV. The *Law of Prevention and Control of HIV/AIDS* provides people living with HIV with the "full right to the freedom of abode and travel." The law states that no person will be placed in isolation, expelled, or "refused abode" based on the HIV status of that person or members of their family. (Cambodia *Law on the Prevention and Control of HIV/AIDS,* July 2002. http://www.ilo.org/public/english/protection/trav/aids/laws/cambodia1.pdf)

In the 2004 *Statement on HIV/AIDS-Related Travel Restrictions,* UNAIDS and IOM recommend voluntary testing for people entering a country. Such testing should only be done with informed consent, and it should include related services, such as counseling both before and after the test and a guarantee of confidentiality. A positive test (or declaration, should a country choose to require it) should not be accompanied by automatic entry restrictions. The statement notes that public health impact is not an appropriate justification for restrictions, and that restrictions for economic reasons should only be imposed after evaluating individual circumstances (UNAIDS & IOM 2004).

References

Aidsnet, *Iceland,* AIDS Info Docu Switzerland (October 14, 2003). http://www.aidsnet.ch/modules.php?name=Content&pa=showpage&pid=121

NAM, *Countries and Their Entry Restrictions,* Aidsmap (NAM April 25 2006). http://www.aidsmap.com/en/docs/C92D5639-E779-44EC-B8F8-0CECCC23275A.asp

Rwebangira, M. K. & M. B. Tungaraza, *Review and Assessment of Laws Affecting HIV/AIDS in Tanzania,* Nov., Chapter 11 (Tanzania Women Lawyers' Association 2003). http://www.policyproject.com/pubs/countryreports/TZlawreview_sumbooklet.pdf http://www.policyproject.com/pubs/countryreports/TZlawreview.pdf (Full report)

UNAIDS & IOM, *Statement on HIV/AIDS-Related Travel Restrictions,* June (UNAIDS & International Organization for Migration 2004). http://www.iom.org.za/Reports/UNAIDS_IOM_StatementOnTravelRestrictions.pdf#search=%22UNAIDS%2FIOM%20Statement %20on%20HIV%2FAIDS-Related%20Travel%20Restrictions%22

UNHCR, *Note on HIV/AIDS and the Protection of Refugees, IDPs and Other Persons of Concern,* April (United Nations High Commissioner for Refugees 2006). http://www.unhcr.org/publ/PUBL/444e20892.pdf

————, *Antiretroviral Medication Policy for Refugees,* January (United Nations High Commissioner for Refugees 2007). http://www.unhcr.org/publ/PUBL/45b479642.pdf

United States Department of State, *Human Immunodeficiency Virus (HIV) Testing Requirements for Entry into Foreign Countries,* March (United States Department of State 2006). http://travel.state.gov/travel/tips/brochures/brochures_1230.html

2.10   Issues at the Border: Refugees and Asylum

The Issue

Many nations have placed restrictions on the entry of HIV-positive persons into their countries (see Topic 2.9). In countries that have enacted such restrictions, these policies may impact the ability of HIV-positive persons to become refugees or receive asylum. HIV-positive persons may be seeking asylum (if they are already in the country) or refugee status (if they seek to enter from abroad) as a direct result of their HIV status. In many areas of the world, PLHIV are faced with oppression, abuse, and discrimination. Additionally, many governments are unable or unwilling to provide effective treatment, including antiretroviral therapy. Because of these concerns, human rights advocates have called for governments to grant asylum or refugee status to people who would otherwise face abuse or persecution in their countries of origin due to their HIV status, or be denied access to HIV treatment due to the circumstances in their home countries. AIDS activists have argued also that people seeking asylum or refugee status on other grounds should not be denied because of their HIV status.

Legal and Policy Considerations

Laws and policies for granting asylum often apply a complicated calculus for determining whether a person meets the criteria to remain in the country. Typically, asylum decisions are fact-specific, based on the discrete circumstances facing a person in their home country. In many countries, asylum will be granted only in cases where the applicant is able to show that there is a high likelihood of abuse, torture, persecution, or significant threats to health if he or she returns home. Similarly, Article 33 of the 1951 *Convention Relating to the Status of Refugees* provides that states must not "expel or return ("refouler") a refugee in any manner whatsoever to the frontiers of territories where his life or freedom would be threatened on account of . . . membership of a particular social group . . ."

Advocates for PLHIV argue that the disease itself should be grounds for asylum in certain circumstances. In many areas of the world, people with HIV are subjected to severe abuse, discrimination, and social ostracism, from both state actors and society in general. Many PLHIV have little or no consistent access to basic health care, much less care for HIV and related infections. Remaining in their country of origin will inevitably result in their deaths. However, with a few exceptions, governments and courts have not been willing to recognize on a consistent basis HIV-status alone as sufficient to qualify for asylum or refugee status. For example, the United States has recognized persecution based on HIV infection as a basis for granting asylum if the applicant can demonstrate that his home government causes "extreme harm" to HIV-positive individuals. However, the United States will not grant asylum solely based on inadequate medical treatment and social ostracism.

In the many states that restrict immigration by people with HIV (see Topic 2.9), refugees and asylum seekers may face significant additional burdens. Some countries refuse to grant asylum or refugee status to people who would otherwise qualify on the basis of their HIV-positive status. For those applicants who have credible fears of persecution in their country of origin, the strict application of national policies prohibiting entry for HIV-positive persons seems particularly inhumane. Under these circumstances, HIV-positive applicants may be prevented from obtaining asylum. More likely, they may not seek asylum, instead opting to live illegally in a country other than their nation of origin. This can have significant adverse effects on their health, since illegal immigrants are less likely to seek health care or acknowledge their HIV infection. Some countries harbor concerns that allowing asylum or refugee status on the basis of HIV status would result in large scale immigration for treatment. Because antiretroviral therapy and other health care services are expensive, this could result in increased utilization of scarce health care resources. This is particularly true for countries that have a policy of providing treatment free of charge for residents who cannot afford it. These countries may also fear that an influx of HIV-positive asylum seekers or refugees would pose a substantial public health threat, although this conclusion is not shared by many public health experts.

Practice Examples

The European Court of Human Rights has ruled that expulsion of an HIV-positive foreign national back to his or her country of origin can violate Article 3 of the European Convention of Human Rights. In one case, a man from St. Kitts was arrested in possession of drugs upon his arrival to the UK. After it was determined that he had AIDS, the court ruled that he could not be sent back to St. Kitts because he would not be able to receive adequate medical treatment there and that the deportation would constitute inhumane treatment by causing imminent death and severe pain and suffering. (*D. v. United Kingdom*, 24 Eur. H.R. Rep. 423 1997)

Several countries in southern Africa—Namibia, South Africa, and Zambia—have pledged to provide refugees the same HIV treatment that is made available to others in the country. Most other southern African countries provide care to refugees unofficially, except for Botswana, which forbids treatment to refugees (UNHCR 2006).

References

Neilson, Victoria, *HIV-Based Persecution in Asylum and Immigration Decisions,* 4 Human Rights 8 (2004).

OHCHR, *Convention Relating to the Status of Refugees, adopted on 28 July 1951,* Art. 43 (Office of the United Nations High Commissioner for Human Rights 1951). http://www.unhchr.ch/html/menu3/b/o_c_ref.htm

Save the Children, *Asylum and Immigration Implications for HIV/AIDS Diagnosis* (Save the Children c.2005, accessed on 02/13/2007). http://www.savethechildren.org.uk/caris/legal/srandi/sr_23.php

UNAIDS & IOM, *Statement on HIV/AIDS-Related Travel Restrictions,* June (UNAIDS & International Organization for Migration 2004). http://www.iom.org.za/Reports/UNAIDS_IOM_StatementOnTravelRestrictions.pdf#search=%22UNAIDS%2FIOM%20Statement%20on%20HIV%2FAIDS-Related%20Travel%20Restrictions%22

UNHCR, *Namibia Joins South Africa and Zambia in Extending HIV/AIDS Treatment to Refugees,* 10 May (United Nations High Commissioner for Refugees 2006). http://www.unhcr.org/cgi-bin/texis/vtx/news/opendoc.htm?tbl=NEWS&id=4461f8d82

UNHCR & UNAIDS, *Strategies to Support the HIV-Related Needs of Refugees and Host Populations,* October (United Nations High Commissioner for Refugees & UNAIDS 2005). http://www.unhcr.org/cgi-bin/texis/vtx/protect/opendoc.pdf?tbl=PROTECTION&id=438ad15d2

2.11   Discrimination in Public and Private Benefits

The Issue

Due to the persistent stigma that often accompanies HIV and AIDS, PLHIV may face discrimination in various contexts. Public and private benefits are no exception. Without adequate legal protection, PLHIV often experience difficulty in obtaining health or life insurance, social security benefits, and credit or other financial services. Also, access to public facilities such as public buildings, parks, hotels, restaurants, buses and trains, and other facilities or areas that are typically open to the general public, should not be denied to PLHIV.

Legal and Policy Considerations

National laws and policies may address discrimination related to benefits, financial services, and access to public accommodations through general anti-discrimination laws. In countries that adopt this approach, the general laws may directly designate antidiscrimination protections for benefits, insurance coverage, or accommodations, guaranteeing that those making decisions in these areas are not discriminating against PLHIV. Legislation and regulations applicable to specific industries, such as insurance or financial services, may also include separate protections against discrimination. For example, in countries where health insurance, life insurance, and other benefits are provided through employers, labor and employment laws may prevent HIV-negative status from being used as a prerequisite for eligibility for insurance or benefits, and may forbid employers and others from sharing information about a person's HIV status with insurers without consent.

A central consideration for policymakers is to find the fair equilibrium between preventing discrimination and allowing the insurance and financial markets to work. Since health directly impacts the insurance scheme, insurance companies need certain private information from the people they insure. Insurers may try to refuse to cover HIV-positive persons or charge an excessively high premium for their coverage. Many countries have found a balance by prohibiting insurance companies from requiring an HIV test or a declaration of HIV status prior to approving insurance coverage, yet still allowing them to make reasonable actuarial decisions. The UNAIDS/OHCHR *International Guidelines on HIV/AIDS and Human Rights* recommend fair and equal treatment of HIV status in insurance: "exemptions for superannuation and life insurance should only relate to reasonable actuarial data, so that HIV/AIDS is not treated differently from analogous medical conditions."

Many people with HIV also have difficulty obtaining social security benefits because many government benefits programs require individuals to have a severe physical or mental health disability that makes it impossible for them to work before they can receive social security. Even if an HIV-positive individual can no longer work, some governments will not uniformly apply benefits, nor will they allow for flexible benefits that address the progressive and intermittent nature of HIV-related disease and AIDS. However, several countries have implemented provisions similar to the recommendations of the ILO's *Code of Practice for HIV/AIDS and the World of Work,* which states that social security and other government-sanctioned benefits should be granted to HIV-positive persons "no less favourably than to workers with other serious illnesses."

Discrimination against PLHIV may occur in financial institutions such as savings and loan companies, credit unions, mortgage banking companies, and credit card issuers. In addition to the potential for discrimination based on generalized animus against PLHIV, financial institutions may not want to loan money or provide credit to persons with HIV or AIDS because the chance of having their money paid back in the future is decreased. Similarly to the areas of insurance and benefits, many national laws prohibit financial institutions from asking about a loan or credit applicant's HIV status, but allow the institution to screen applicants based on other factors. Pursuant to these provisions, the loan applicant with HIV must be treated equally to other applicants who are similarly situated.

Finally, people living with HIV may experience discrimination in everyday life when they try to access public accommodations or facilities. Public accommodations include any privately-owned businesses that provide goods or services to the general public, such as restaurants, hotels, retail stores, schools, theaters, hospitals, health clinics, and personal service providers, as well as public spaces and facilities like parks, libraries, and public transportation. In many countries, anti-discrimination laws prohibit differential treatment based upon HIV status in this context as well.

Practice Examples

Article 40 of the Cambodia *Law on the Prevention and Control of HIV/AIDS* states: "Discrimination against persons with HIV/AIDS in access to all credits or loans services including health, accident and life insurance, upon such concerned person who meets all technical criteria as other uninfected citizens, is strictly prohibited."

In South Africa, the *Medical Schemes Act,* No 131 of 1998 provides that a registered medical aid scheme may not unfairly discriminate directly or indirectly against its members on the basis of their state of health, including HIV status. The Act prescribes minimum benefits for HIV infection as well. In addition, the South African *Charter of Rights on AIDS and HIV* states that "Persons with AIDS or HIV should have equal access to public benefits and opportunities, and HIV testing should not be required as a precondition for eligibility to such advantages." (http://alp.org.za/images/upload/3rdAids%20finalss%20append.pdf)

South Africa's Promotion of Equality and Prevention of Unfair Discrimination Act, 2000 provides in its Schedule an illustrative list of unfair practices, including discrimination with respect to health care services and benefits, housing, accommodation, land and property, and insurance services. (http://www.acts .co.za/prom_of_ equality)

In the Philippines, the *AIDS Prevention and Control Act 1998,* Section 39, provides substantial protection against discrimination: "All credit and loan services, including health, accident and life insurance shall not be denied to a person on the basis of his/her actual, perceived or suspected HIV status: *Provided,* that the person with HIV has not concealed or misrepresented the fact to the insurance company upon application. Extension and continuation of credit and loan shall likewise not be denied solely on the basis of said health condition."

References

Canadian HIV/AIDS Legal Network, *International News: UK Doctors Given New Guidance on Revealing HIV Test and Sexual History to Insurers,* 8(1) HIV/AIDS Policy and Law Rev. (2003). http://www.aidslaw.ca/publications/publicationsdocEN.php?ref=248

Government of South Africa, *Promotion of Equality and Prevention of Unfair Discrimination Act* (Government of South Africa 2000). http://www.acts.co.za/prom_of_equality

ILO, *An ILO Code of Practice on HIV/AIDS and the World of Work* (International Labour Organization 2001). http://www.ilo.org/public/english/protection/trav/aids/code/languages/hiv_a4_e.pdf

UNAIDS & OHCHR, *International Guidelines on HIV/AIDS and Human Rights*, 2006 Consolidated version (UNAIDS & Office of the United Nations High Commissioner for Human Rights 2006). http://data.unaids.org/Publications/IRC-pub07/JC1252-InternGuidelines_en.pdf?preview=true

SECTION 3

Disclosure and Exposure

3.1 Duty to Disclose HIV Status to Partner

The Issue

Individuals who are aware that they are infected with HIV are ethically obligated to attempt to protect others with whom they engage in sexual contact or injecting drug use from infection. But is there a legal duty of disclosure? Disclosure of one's HIV-positive status may infringe upon individual privacy, and elicit fears of social rejection, retaliatory violence by partners, and societal discrimination. Partners may also have an obligation to take steps to protect themselves from infection (or reinfection), including using a condom or sterile injecting equipment.

Legal and Policy Considerations

Misrepresentation may occur either by (1) withholding information about one's serostatus, or (2) intentionally lying about it. The latter, aside from practical issues of proof of lying ("he said, she said") and resulting harm, does not pose conceptual difficulties under general civil and criminal fraud or similar statutes. However, if a person does not know for sure that he or she is HIV-positive, but knows that there may be a chance of being infected, does nondisclosure of that fact amount to misrepresentation? Given the grave consequences of contracting HIV, public health considerations could lead to an affirmative answer. However, any person who ever had risky, unprotected sex might then become potentially liable. This would be an impractical and unwarranted extension of the concept of misrepresentation and might lead to liability by affiliation especially for members of high risk groups such as men who have sex with men or injecting drug users.

Legal and ethical principles of informed consent mandate that individuals at risk of concealed harms be made aware of such risks. Accordingly, the defense that the sexual or needle-sharing partner consented to the act would not normally be available in cases of intentional misrepresentation, especially if appropriate measures to avoid the risk of harm were not taken. The absence of informed consent may also have other legal consequences; it may, for example, be grounds for annulment of marriages.

A criminal statute requiring disclosure of one's HIV-positive status to partners may be viewed as an effective tool to protect public health if it is believed that many HIV-positive persons would not take precautions to prevent transmission and might otherwise choose not to inform their partners. Many governments have adopted such laws. However, such statutes have been criticized as infringing individual privacy, placing vulnerable persons at risk, and being difficult to implement. Importantly, they may undermine a country's efforts to encourage voluntary counseling and testing: individuals who know they may be at risk of having contracted the virus may avoid getting tested, further driving the epidemic underground. In addition, these laws present difficult issues in the courtroom relating to burden of proof and consent. The UNAIDS & OHCHR *International Guidelines on HIV/AIDS and Human Rights* and the UNAIDS & IPU *Handbook for Legislators* advise against the enactment of HIV-specific criminal statutes in this area.

UNAIDS and WHO encourage voluntary disclosure and ethical partner counseling. These programs rely on professional counseling of HIV-positive clients to encourage them to notify partners and get these partners to seek counseling (see Topic 1.4). If there should be repeated refusal by the HIV-positive client to notify his or her partners, the health care professional/counselor should be empowered to notify and counsel the partner(s) after weighing the harms and benefits to all parties (see Topics 1.5, 1.6). These voluntary programs, often organized or operated by governmental public health entities, tend to be less infringing of individual privacy, contribute to a culture of openness about HIV, and may help improve the health of the infected individual and his or her partners through early notification and opportunities to connect exposed individuals to other public health interventions.

Practice Examples

A New Zealand court (in 2005) ruled that persons with HIV have a legal duty to exercise reasonable care to avoid spreading the virus, which can be satisfied by the individual's use of a condom during vaginal intercourse. (E.J. Bernard. "Groundbreaking New Zealand ruling finds condom use eliminates HIV disclosure requirement." October 9, 2005. http://www.aidsmap.com/en/news/99FCF282-21EF-4ED5-99FC-B3A9E2E1A110.asp)

In *R. v. Cuerrier,* the Canadian Supreme Court held that failure to disclose HIV status can constitute assault and fraud in situations where significant risk of HIV transmission is possible. (*R. v. Cuerrier,* 2 S.C.R. 371 (1998). http://www.lexum.umontreal.ca. The response of the Canadian HIV/AIDS Legal Network ("Supreme Court Ruling Will Harm HIV Prevention," Press Release, Sept. 3, 1998) may be found at http://www.aidslaw.ca/publications/mediaEN.php?l_id=1)

Examples of laws requiring disclosure to sexual partners while providing a facilitating role for health care workers/counselors:

- Philippine AIDS Prevention and Control Act of 1998 (RA 8504), Section 34, and Rules and Regulations Implementing the *Philippine AIDS Prevention and Control Act of 1998* (RA 8504), Section 45. (http://www.doh.gov.ph/aids/publication.htm)

- Republica Dominicana, *Ley No. 55-93 Sobre el SIDA,* Art. 21. (http://www
.suprema.gov.do/pdf/leyes/Ley%20numero%2055%20sida.pdf)

In India:

- In matrimonial law, courts have held that "concealment of serious disease"
amounts to fraud and is sufficient grounds to annul marriages. *Hindu Marriage Act of 1955* § 23(bb). (http://indiacode.nic.in)
- Under tort law, an HIV-infected individual who withholds information
about his or her status and either causes or exposes a partner to injury, without necessarily transmitting HIV, can be held liable for battery, assault, negligence, and fraud (including the "active concealment of a fact by one
having knowledge or belief of the fact") under Chapter VI § 25 (iii) of
the *Special Marriage Act of 1954* with reference to Chapter II § 17(2) of the
Indian Contract Act of 1872. (http://indiacode.nic.in)

A U.S. judge sentenced a man to 44 years in prison for failing to disclose his
HIV status to at least 11 female partners before engaging in consensual sex. *State
of Idaho v. Mubita,* Second Judicial District, May 31, 2006, as reported by
D. Johnson. *Lewiston Morning Tribune,* May 2006; 1C. (http://www.lmtribune
.com/05262006/northwes/northwes.php)

References

Dwyer, John M., *Legislating AIDS Away: the Limited Role of Legal Persuasion in Minimizing
the Spread of the Human Immunodeficiency Virus,* 9 J. Contemp. Health L. & Policy 167
(1993).

Hodge, James G. Jr. & Lawrence O. Gostin, *Handling Cases of Willful Exposure through HIV
Partner Counseling and Referral Services,* 22 Women's Rights Law Reporter 45–62 (2001).

Lawyers' Collective, HIV/AIDS Unit, *Positive Dialogue,* 17 Newsletter, June (Lawyers'
Collective 2004). http://www.lawyerscollective.org/lc_hivaids/publications/newsletters/
newsletter_17.pdf

Niccolai, L. M., D. Dorst, L. Myers & P. J. Kissinger, *Disclosure of HIV Status to Sexual Partners: Predictors and Temporal Patterns,* 26 Sexually Transmitted Diseases 281–85 (1999).

Russell, S., *Shift in AIDS Prevention Strategy: Emphasis Now on Accountability of Those
Infected* (San Francisco Chronicle, September 21, 2003). http://www.aegis.org/NEWS/
SC/2003/SC030908.html

UNAIDS, *Opening Up the HIV/AIDS Epidemic: Guidance on Encouraging Beneficial Disclosure, Ethical Partner Counseling and Appropriate Use of HIV Case-Reporting* (UNAIDS
2000). http://data.unaids.org/Publications/IRC-pub05/JC488-OpenUp_en.pdf

———, *Criminal Law, Public Health, and HIV Transmission: A Policy Options Paper*
(UNAIDS 2002).

UNAIDS & IPU, *Handbook for Legislators on HIV/AIDS, Law and Human Rights: Action to Combat HIV/AIDS in View of Its Devastating Human, Economic, and Social Impact* (UNAIDS & Inter-Parliamentary Union 1999). http://www.ipu.org/PDF/publications/aids_en.pdf

UNAIDS & OHCHR, *International Guidelines on HIV/AIDS and Human Rights,* 2006 Consolidated version (UNAIDS & Office of the United Nations High Commissioner for Human Rights 2006). http://data.unaids.org/Publications/IRC-pub07/JC1252-InternGuidelines_en.pdf?preview=true

Weait, Matthew & Yusef Azad, *The Criminalization of HIV Transmission in England and Wales: Questions of Law and Policy,* 10(2) HIV/AIDS Policy and Law Rev. 1 (2005). http://www.aidslaw.ca/publications/publicationsdocEN.php?ref=224

3.2 Negligent or Willful Exposure or Transmission

The Issue

An individual who knowingly exposes an unknowing partner to HIV may negligently spread the virus without any malicious intent. A person infected with HIV may take precautions to prevent its spread, only to have those precautions fail due to his own negligence. Attaching criminal or other sanctions to individuals in these cases may be antithetical to public health objectives. Others, however, may willfully or recklessly attempt to spread HIV. In these cases, HIV-positive individuals may intentionally engage in risky sexual or drug-sharing behaviors to harm an unknowing partner. Alternatively, the individual may act in a reckless manner from which criminal or malicious intent may be presumed. Often some level of civil or criminal culpability is assigned to individuals in these cases, especially when exposure leads to transmission.

Legal and Policy Considerations

Laws and policies that criminalize negligent or willful exposure seek to deter individuals whose actions lead to exposure of others to HIV and potential transmission. The legal ramifications of exposing an uninfected individual to HIV differ depending on (a) intent; and (b) whether transmission of HIV occurs, although each element can be difficult to prove legally or epidemiologically.

Intent is tied to the type and severity of the offense and punishment. The intentional exposure of another to a communicable disease is deemed a crime in most jurisdictions under general criminal law (e.g., manslaughter, assault and battery, reckless endangerment, or attempts of each of these crimes). As noted by UNAIDS, addressing the relatively few numbers of cases of intentional exposure or transmission of HIV through general criminal laws is preferable to crafting STD- or HIV-specific offenses given the potential for targeted enforcement and discrimination. Also, HIV-specific criminal statutes may discourage voluntary testing and thereby counteract governments' prevention efforts. Still, some jurisdictions have created specific criminal sanctions for intentional HIV offenses.

Transmission of HIV is not always a necessary element of criminal charges or civil causes of action. Yet when transmission actually occurs, the severity of criminal charges or civil claims may be augmented. For example, willful exposure of HIV may result in a criminal charge of assault; willful exposure resulting in transmission may sustain a charge of attempted voluntary manslaughter or even murder (if the partner dies as a result of exposure to HIV).

Practice Example

California lawmakers have made it a crime to knowingly expose a sexual partner to HIV, but require that the individual acted with "specific intent" to spread the disease to his or her partner or partners. The crime is punishable by eight years in prison (Kaiser Family Foundation 2003).

References

Canadian HIV/AIDS.Legal Network, *Legal and Ethical Issues Raised by HIV/AIDS,* 1 Literature Review 3 (Canadian HIV/AIDS Legal Network 1999). http://www.aidslaw.ca/publications/interfaces/downloadFile.php?ref=18#search=%22Legal%20and%20ethical%20issues%20raised%20by%20HIV%2FAIDS%20%E2%80%93%20Literature%20Reviw%201%2C%203.%20Ontario%22

Hodge, James G. Jr. & Lawrence O. Gostin, *Handling Cases of Willful Exposure through HIV Partner Counseling and Referral Services,* 22 Women's Rights Law Reporter 45–62 (2001).

Kaiser Family Foundation, *California Law against Knowingly Transmitting HIV Too Narrow, Prosecutors Say,* Kaiser Daily HIV/AIDS Report, September 10 (Kaiser Family Foundation 2003). www.Kaisernetwork.org/daily_reports/print_report.cfm?DR_ID=19777&dr_cat=1

MAHA, *Switzerland: A New HIV Transmission Conviction Exposes the Link between Racism and Public Health,* August 1 (Migrants Contre le SIDA 1996). http://www.survivreausida.net/a2634

UNAIDS, *Criminal Law, Public Health and HIV Transmission: A Policy Options Paper* (UNAIDS 2002). http://data.unaids.org/Publications/IRC-pub02/JC733-CriminalLaw_en.pdf#search=%22UNAIDS.%20Criminal%20Law%2C%20Public%20Health%20and%20HIV%20Transmission%3A%20A%20Policy%20Options%20Paper%22

SECTION 4

Injecting Drug Use

4.1 Access to Clean Needles and Drug Paraphernalia Laws

The Issue

Injecting drug use is a main pathway for the spread of HIV. While globally, most HIV is transmitted sexually, an estimated 10% is transmitted through injecting drug use (IDU). In some countries in Asia and Europe, the majority of HIV infections are due to IDU. Once HIV enters a population of intravenous drug users, it spreads quickly. For example, between 1993 and 1998, prevalence of HIV among injecting drug users in Manipur, India skyrocketed from 1 to 60 percent. From the IDU community, HIV then spreads more widely through sexual transmission.

Injecting drugs is an efficient way to transmit the HIV virus. A user may draw blood back into the syringe and re-inject the mixture of blood and trace amount of drugs to ensure more of the drug is injected. Even using a syringe without this practice can cause contamination, and a combination of drug-using culture and perceived necessity may lead to the reuse of needles. Scientists have detected viable HIV in syringes stored at room temperature for up to four weeks.

Legal and Policy Considerations

While reusing needles is dangerous, some countries have laws in place that hamper access to clean needles. In some countries, syringes cannot be obtained at a pharmacy without a prescription. Additionally, in many countries, drug paraphernalia laws make possessing syringes for drug use unlawful. The WHO has found that such legislation is a barrier to effective HIV prevention. In fact, there is evidence that restricting access to injecting paraphernalia inadvertently increases the incidence of HIV infection.

Access to sterile needles can be provided through deregulation of their possession, where they are regulated. Where buying needles is legal, drug paraphernalia laws that criminalize possession of needles when intended for drug use deter drug users from purchasing them. Police may arrest, detain, or extract bribes from people solely because they are carrying a syringe. Drug users have cited fear of arrest in numerous studies as the reason they do not carry clean needles. In places where harm reduction programs exist (including needle exchange, discussed in Topic 4.2), injecting drug users may shy away from the access provided fearing arrest. This is apparently the case even where government officials and police have agreed to turn a blind eye to injecting drug users entering and exiting facilities.

Therefore many AIDS activists and public health officials urge countries to decriminalize the purchase and possession of syringes and related material as a crucial tool to slow the spread of HIV among injecting drug users as well as the population at large.

Practice Examples

Some of the most restrictive legislation regarding purchasing of syringes exists in the United States. In July 1992, the state of Connecticut passed a law permitting the purchase and possession of up to ten syringes without a prescription and made parallel changes in its paraphernalia law. Following the legislative changes, there was an increase in the number of syringes sold in pharmacies, self-reported needle sharing declined, as did the incidence and prevalence of HIV. (Conn. Gen. Stat. § 21a-65 2006)

As pharmacies are often closed at night, some countries have experimented with the installation of syringe vending machines, to make needles available at all times. In New South Wales, Australia, for example, the *Needle and Syringe Program Policy and Guidelines* provide for multiple points of access to clean needles including vending machines, pharmacies, and centers designed to provide needles along with other health and drug cessation services. (http://www.health.nsw.gov.au/policies/pd/2006/PD2006_037.html)

The Canadian HIV/AIDS Legal Network has drafted *Model Legislation Addressing the HIV Epidemic among People Who Use Drugs*. The model legislation includes provisions for establishing a needle exchange program, as well as citations to other national laws regarding such programs. The various modules of the model legislation can be accessed at www.aidslaw.ca/drugpolicy

References

Burris, Scott & Daniel Villena, *Adapting to the Reality of HIV: Difficult Policy Choices in Russia, China and India,* 31 Human Rights (2004). http://www.abanet.org/irr/hr/fall04/reality.htm

Canadian HIV/AIDS Legal Network, *Model Legislation Addressing the HIV Epidemic among People Who Use Drugs,* draft (Canadian HIV/AIDS Legal Network 2006). http://www.aidslaw.ca/publications/interfaces/downloadFile.php?ref=141#search=%22Model%20Legislation%20addressing%20the%20HIV%20epidemic%20among%20People%20who%20Use%20Drugs%22

Gostin, Lawrence O., Zita Lazzarini, K. Flaherty, & T. S. Jones, *Prevention of HIV/AIDS and Other Blood-Borne Diseases among Injecting Drug Users: A National Survey on the Regulation of Syringes and Needles,* 277(1) JAMA 53–62 (1997).

Hammett, Theodore M., Nicholas A. Bartlett, Yi Chen, et al., *Law Enforcement Influences on HIV Prevention for Injecting Drug Users,* 16 Int'l J. of Drug Policy 235 (2005).

Institute of Medicine, *Preventing HIV Infection among Injecting Drug Users in High Risk Countries* (Institute of Medicine 2006). http://www.iom.edu/CMS/3783/30188/37071.aspx

Lawyers' Collective, *Legislating an Epidemic: HIV/AIDS in India,* Chapter 5 (Universal Law Publishing Co. Pvt. Ltd. 2003).

UNAIDS, *Joint UNAIDS Statement on HIV Prevention and Care Strategies for Drug Users* (UNAIDS 2005). http://data.unaids.org/UNA-docs/CCO_IDUPolicy_en.pdf

WHO, *Policy Brief: Provision of Sterile Injecting Equipment to Reduce HIV Transmission* (World Health Organization 2004). http://www.wpro.who.int/NR/rdonlyres/BA463DB4-2390-4964-9D86-11CBABCC9DA9/0/provisionofsterileen.pdf

———, *Evidence for Action Technical Papers: Effectiveness of Sterile Needle and Syringe Programming in Reducing HIV/AIDS among Injecting Drug Users* (World Health Organization 2004). http://www.who.int/hiv/pub/prev_care/en/effectivenesssterileneedle.pdf

4.2   Needle/Syringe Exchange Programs

The Issue

Needle exchange programs (also known as NEPs, or syringe exchange programs, SEPs) allow injecting drug users to receive a clean needle and syringe in exchange for turning in a used set. These programs are often controversial, as they may be illegal under a country's drug laws. In addition, communities may worry that exchange programs give citizens the idea that drug use is permissible, increase drug use, or devote resources to unpopular sectors of society. Needle exchange programs have been extraordinarily successful in minimizing the transmission of HIV. In a review of more than 200 studies, the WHO found that the "HIV infection rate had declined by an average of 18.6% annually in 36 cities with needle and syringe programmes, whereas it had increased by an average of 8.1% annually in 67 cities lacking such programmes."

Needle exchange programs have also proven to be extremely cost effective, especially when the long-term consequences of transmission of HIV and other blood-borne diseases are considered. Importantly, studies have found no evidence that exchange programs increase illicit drug use, increase injecting frequency among users, or recruit new users. Consequently, NEPs have been successful at slowing the transmission of HIV among injecting drug users and the rest of the population.

Legal and Policy Considerations

Exchange programs have proved to be an important strategy for limiting the transmission of HIV among injecting drug users and the nondrug using population. Several countries, including Australia, the United States, Canada, Brazil, Nepal, and the Russian Federation, have implemented exchange programs (although sometimes on a small scale). These programs have been authorized under law, in some cases as exceptions to existing drug laws.

Needle exchange programs can require users to turn in old needles, thereby reducing the quantity of contaminated equipment in the community. However, many programs do not require users to turn in needles to receive replacements. Especially where law proscribes the possession of drug paraphernalia, injecting drug users may be reluctant to travel with used needles. Programs may also give needle vouchers, which can be used at pharmacies to obtain clean needles, or permit secondary distribution of needles by the injecting drug users served. In some exchange programs, condoms and ampoules of water are also supplied. Exchange programs can be stationary or mobile, the choice depending on which will serve more people. Needle exchange programs have been introduced in some prisons, where rates of transmission are high and drug use continues even under difficult circumstances. Health interventions for prison populations also serve broader public health goals, as the overwhelming majority of prisoners will return to the general public. Needle exchange programs can also benefit injecting drug users by creating a potential for them to request or receive help or education through the exchange workers.

In order for NEPs to be effective, laws need to ensure that all of those involved are protected from arrest, including exchange workers, pharmacists, medical practitioners, and users. Laws that criminalize "facilitation" or "incitement" of drug use should exclude all aspects of needle exchange programs. Education and provision of information about the exchange must also be lawful. Users must not be made criminally liable for possession of syringes or of trace amounts of drugs found in used syringes that are going to be turned in. Records of syringe exchanges as well as exchange workers must be protected from subpoena by police and being used as evidence in drug-related legal proceedings. If injecting drug users fear that using an exchange program could lead to their arrest, the program will not be successful. Several countries also incorporate training of police to ensure that they do not harass users of syringe exchange programs or use the sites to gather information for criminal proceedings.

Practice Examples

In the 1990s, Ukraine realized the need to reform its law to allow for harm reduction approaches, including needle exchange. The government established a National AIDS Committee composed of experts and studied the legislation of other countries to determine best practices. In 1998, the law was amended to allow for needle exchange programs (Art. 4) and to abolish mandatory HIV testing of injecting drug users. Lawmakers and the general public had to be convinced that legalizing NEPs would not promote drug use. (*The Law on Acquired Immune Deficiency Syndrome (AIDS) Prevention and Social Protection of Population,* 155/98-VR, March 3, 1998, described in UNDCP & UNAIDS, *Drug Abuse and HIV/AIDS: Lessons Learned,* 2002, at 71)

The Canadian HIV/AIDS Legal Network has drafted *Model Legislation addressing the HIV Epidemic among People who Use Drugs.* The draft legislation includes provisions for establishing a needle exchange program, as well as citations to other national laws regarding such programs (Canadian HIV/AIDS Legal Network 2006).

Finally, some countries are experimenting with supervised drug use facilities, where people can use drugs safely, under the supervision of health care professionals (J. Kimber et al. 2003).

References

Canadian HIV/AIDS Legal Network, *Model Law on Drug Use and HIV/AIDS* (Canadian HIV/AIDS Legal Network 2006). http://www.aidslaw.ca/publications/publicationsEN .php?t_id=5&l_id=1&sort=date

———, *Prison Needle Exchange: Lessons from a Comprehensive Review of International Evidence and Experience* (2nd ed., Canadian HIV/AIDS Legal Network 2006). http://www .aidslaw.ca/prisons

Hammett, Theodore M., Nicholas A. Bartlett, Yi Chen, et al., *Law Enforcement Influences on HIV Prevention for Injecting Drug Users,* 16 Int'l J. of Drug Policy 235 (2005).

Institute of Medicine, *Preventing HIV Infection among Injecting Drug Users in High Risk Countries* (Institute of Medicine 2006). http://www.iom.edu/CMS/3783/30188/37071.aspx

Kimber, J., et al., *Drug Consumption Facilities: An Update since 2000,* 227 Drug and Alcohol Review (2003).

Pearshouse, Richard, Richard Elliott, Joanne Csete & Glenn Betteridge, *Barriers to Harm Reduction: Legal Issues Related to Assisted Injection at Safe Injection Facilities* (Canadian HIV/AIDS Legal Network 2006). http://www.aidslaw.ca/publications/interfaces/ downloadFile.php?ref=660

UNAIDS, *Joint UNAIDS Statement on HIV Prevention and Care Strategies for Drug Users* (UNAIDS 2005). http://data.unaids.org/UNA-docs/CCO_IDUPolicy_en.pdf

UNDCP & UNAIDS, *Drug Abuse and HIV/AIDS: Lessons Learned* (United Nations International Drug Control Programme & UNAIDS 2002).

WHO, *Policy Brief: Provision of Sterile Injecting Equipment to Reduce HIV Transmission* (World Health Organization 2004). http://www.wpro.who.int/NR/rdonlyres/BA463DB4-2390-4964-9D86-11CBABCC9DA9/0/provisionofsterileen.pdf

———, *Evidence for Action Technical Papers: Effectiveness of Sterile Needle and Syringe Programming in Reducing HIV/AIDS among Injecting Drug Users* (World Health Organization 2004). http://www.who.int/hiv/pub/prev_care/en/effectivenesssterileneedle.pdf

———, *Status Paper on Prisons, Drugs and Harm Reduction* (World Health Organization 2005). www.euro.who.int/document/e85877.pdf

4.3   Drug Substitution Programs

The Issue

Drug substitution programs have been widely used to treat injecting drug users for their addictions. Drug substitution programs (or substitution maintenance therapies) are among the most effective treatments for opioid dependency. Opioids, including opium, morphine, codeine, and heroin, are commonly injected. Drug substitution programs provide a prescribed psychoactive substance, related to the one producing dependence, under medical supervision. The substitute drug often works by reducing the craving for the illicit drug without providing a "high" or other euphoric effect. Such programs are controversial, as injecting drug users are generally a very stigmatized population. However, evidence demonstrates that these policies can be effective at reducing injecting drug use and therefore the associated transmission of HIV.

Legal and Policy Considerations

Drug substitution therapy has been implemented in various forms in many countries. Some countries have authorized drug substitution programs within more general legislation for illicit drug regulation. Another approach has been to pass legislation or enact policies that specifically authorize drug substitution. These provisions may even dictate specific drugs to be used and detailed procedures for oversight. Many substitution therapy programs are designed using the principles of good medical practice. Evidence-based guidelines include eligibility requirements for the program, contraindications, best practices in clinical management, and relevant government regulations. Regulations can be aimed at improving the quality of treatment, and not be so restrictive as to deny access to individuals who would benefit from treatment. Medical issues such as maximum doses or maximum length of treatments should be determined by a practitioner's clinical judgment, and based on an individualized assessment of a patient. Registering and/or accrediting treatment providers can help to ensure quality of service and reduce the risk of prescribed medicines reaching illicit channels.

Treatment with a drug substitute has been shown to be effective in curtailing drug use as well as reducing the incidence of HIV. Even so, programs for the provision of substitute drugs can be highly contentious. According to a position paper produced jointly by the World Health Organization, United Nations Office on Drugs and Crime, and the Joint United Nations Programme on HIV/AIDS (UNAIDS), substitution therapy "is in line with the 1961 and 1971 Conventions on narcotic drugs and psychotropic substances" (see Topic 4.4).

Effective treatment of drug addiction can prevent HIV transmission in a variety of ways. Reduced use of needles—especially contaminated needles—means a reduced incidence of HIV transmission. In addition, treatment can decrease criminal behavior, increase the potential for legal employment, and increase the efficacy of treatment for HIV because drug-free individuals are more likely to adhere to treatment regimens. Further, stopping drug injecting may slow the progression of HIV. Injecting drug users who enter and remain in treatment are up to six times less likely to become infected with HIV.

Methadone is the drug most often used in substitution therapy, and its effectiveness has been widely studied. In 2005 WHO added methadone to its List of Essential Medicines. Other drugs used for therapy include buprenorphine, levo alpha acetyl methadol (LAAM), dihydrocodeine, laudanum, and diacetylmorphine (heroin, assessed in the Netherlands and Switzerland for treatment of those severely dependent). Because treatment is safe and effective, it is widely considered a very cost effective alternative to imprisonment or continued illegal drug use. However, despite its efficacy and public health benefits, methadone programs are legal in only 19 low- and middle-income countries.

Opponents of drug substitution programs often object to the provision of drugs to addicted persons and the focus on treatment rather than punishment for illicit drug use. However, pure criminal justice interventions (imprisonment or other sanctions, without dependence treatment) have been shown to have limited impact on drug injecting behavior, and recidivism among injecting drug users is high.

Practice Examples

In some countries, legislation is enacted to try to control the use of all drugs. Usually through regulation, drugs are classified in different schedules, according to the extent of regulation on their use. In the United States, Canada, and the United Kingdom, methadone is classified among drugs with a high potential for abuse or addiction, but that have medicinal use. This classification triggers the requirement that the drug be prescribed by a physician as well as other constraints.

Other countries have drafted regulations specific to the use of substitution therapy. Estonian regulations have several requirements, including that the medicine be prescribed by a doctor or psychiatrist, review of the treatment every six months, and reporting requirements. It is worth noting that where substitution therapy is too constrictively regulated, there may not be sufficient resources for those seeking treatment. A translation of Estonia's regulations is available at http://www.ceehrn.org/EasyCEE/sys/files/Estonian%20national%20guidelines.doc.

References

Aro, Tiiu, *On Providing Drug Users (DUs) with Maintenance and Detoxification Treatment in Various Phases* (Ministry of Social Affairs, Estonia 1998). http://www.ceehrn.org/EasyCEE/sys/files/Estonian%20national%20guidelines.doc

Butler, William, *HIV/AIDS and Drug Misuse in Russia: Harm Reduction Programmes and the Russian Legal System,* Chapter 10 (Family Health International, London, 2003).

Institute of Medicine, *Preventing HIV Infection among Injecting Drug Users in High Risk Countries* (Institute of Medicine 2006). http://www.iom.edu/CMS/3783/30188/37071.aspx

International Harm Reduction Development, Open Society Institute, *Protecting the Human Rights of Injection Drug Users: The Impact of HIV and AIDS* (Open Society Institute 2005).

Prasada Rao, J. V. R., *Plenary Speech* (XVII International Harm Reduction Conference, Vancouver, April 30, 2006). http://data.unaids.org/pub/Speech/2006/20060508_SP_Vancouver_Rao_en.pdf

UNAIDS, *Drug Use and HIV/AIDS: UNAIDS Statement Presented at the United Nations General Assembly Special Session on Drugs* (UNAIDS 1999).

———, *Joint UNAIDS Statement on HIV Prevention and Care Strategies for Drug Users* (UNAIDS 2005). http://data.unaids.org/UNA-docs/CCO_IDUPolicy_en.pdf

WHO, *Policy Brief: Antiretroviral Therapy and Injecting Drug Users* (World Health Organization 2005). http://www.wpro.who.int/NR/rdonlyres/539F9FB1-0801-49B9-BAFF-B6FF88EF6583/0/antiretroviraltherapy.pdf

WHO, UNODC & UNAIDS, *Position Paper: Substitution Maintenance Therapy in the Management of Opioid Dependence and HIV/AIDS Prevention* (World Health Organization, United Nations Office on Drugs and Crime & UNAIDS 2004).

4.4   International Drug Conventions: Punitive v. Public Health Approach

The Issue

The framework for international treaties regarding drug control is law enforcement, not public health. The goal is to eliminate illicit drugs mainly through punitive responses towards traffickers, sellers, buyers, and users. Extensive prison sentences are the lynchpin of this framework, and treatment for addiction and safe injecting of drugs are not priorities. As a result, the primary bodies responsible for implementing and monitoring drug policy have been reluctant to endorse proven harm reduction strategies. Even so, it can be argued that countries can legally implement harm reduction strategies consistent with the drug control conventions.

Legal and Policy Considerations

The 1961 *Single Convention on Narcotic Drugs* as amended in 1972 classifies drugs on the basis of danger and medical benefit, and limits the use, trade, and production of drugs to medical and scientific purposes through international cooperation. The convention identifies methadone, the most prevalently used drug for assisting heroin addicts in drug substitution programs, as a "schedule 1" drug to which access should be strictly limited. The *Convention on Psychotropic Substances* (1971) classifies additional drugs (primarily psychotropics that became popular in the 1960s and 1970s). A 13 member International Narcotics Control Board (INCB) is tasked with monitoring country compliance with the treaties. The 1988 *Convention against Illicit Traffic in Narcotic Drugs and Psychotropic Substances* added precursor chemicals (used for manufacture of illicit drugs) to the list of controlled substances, and sought to regulate the financial aspects of the drug trade, including money laundering and seizure of assets. In addition, signatories to the 1988 Convention are required to criminalize "possession, purchase or cultivation of narcotic or psychotropic drugs for personal consumption."

There is considerable debate regarding whether harm reduction techniques, such as needle exchange, the prescription of methadone or heroin to addicts, or supervised drug consumption facilities, are compatible with the conventions. National governments have used the international drug control treaties to justify punitive drug policies and the lack of harm reduction strategies that have been proven to reduce the incidence of HIV. On the other hand, many see the covenants as including the necessary flexibility to accommodate harm reduction strategies. There is discretion under the treaties to determine what constitutes "medical" or "scientific" use. Countries have maintained that harm reduction strategies fall under this category, and are consistent with the conventions.

The *Single Convention* also provides for the option of offering "either as an alternative to conviction or punishment or in addition to conviction or punishment, . . . treatment, education, after-care, rehabilitation and social reintegration . . ." (Single Convention, Art. 36(1)(b)). While the 1988 Convention requires criminalization of possession and purchase of drugs, it does not specify what penalties are required. Thus, some commentators have argued that counseling would be adequate, or that, under the terms of the treaty, penalties are not necessary if they contravene the state's constitution or basic legal principles.

Practice Examples

In practice, and under pressure from the United States, the INCB and the Commission on Narcotic Drugs (an elected body that guides U.N. drug policy) have had difficulty envisioning public health harm reduction strategies as consistent with the conventions. Generally speaking, those that believe in the law enforcement framework think that harm reduction strategies facilitate drug use and possession, incite drug use, or facilitate or aid drug trafficking. (Though, as noted in Topic 4.2, the evidence does not support this view.)

In 2003, the INCB stated that substitution and maintenance treatment did "not constitute any breach of treaty provisions, whatever substance may be used for such treatment in line with established national sound medical practice." (INCB Report 2003, para. 222. http://www.incb.org/incb/en/annual_report_2003.html) However, more recently, the Board has expressed concern over the prescription of heroin for medical purposes. See INCB 2004 report at para. 201.

There is some evidence that international drug control policy is moving in the direction of acceptance of harm reduction techniques. With respect to needle exchange programs, a recent resolution by the Commission on Narcotic Drugs stopped short of explicitly advocating such programs, and instead noted "the need for Governments to adopt measures aimed at the reduction of needle-sharing among injecting drug users in order to control the spread of HIV/AIDS by that means," but kept in mind "that any prophylactic measures should not promote or facilitate drug abuse." Resolution 49/4, Responding to the Prevalence of HIV/AIDS and Other Blood-Borne Disease among Drug Users, 2006.

References

Aoyagi, Melissa, *Beyond Punitive Prohibition: Liberalizing the Dialogue on International Drug Policy,* 37 NYU J. Int'l L. & Pol. 555 (2005).

INCD, *Report of the International Narcotics Control Board for 2003* (International Narcotics Control Board 2003). http://www.incb.org/incb/en/annual_report_2003.html

———, *Report of the International Narcotics Control Board for 2004* (International Narcotics Control Board 2004). http://www.incb.org/incb/en/annual_report_2004.html

Room, Robin, *Trends and Issues in the International Drug Control System, Vienna 2003,* 37 Journal of Psychoactive Drugs 373–83 (2005).

UNCND, *Report of the Executive Director: Strengthening Strategies Regarding the Prevention of HIV/AIDS in the Context of Drug Abuse,* E/CN.7/2004/3 (United Nations Commission on Narcotic Drugs 2004). http://daccessdds.un.org/doc/UNDOC/GEN/V04/502/27/PDF/V0450227.pdf?OpenElement

Wolfe, Daniel, and Kasia Malinowska-Sempruch, *Illicit Drug Policies and the Global HIV Epidemic: Effects of UN and National Government Approaches* (Open Society Institute, New York 2004).

SECTION 5

Sex Work

5.1   Criminal Statutes on Sex Work

The Issue

Sex work may be nearly universal, but is often illegal and therefore pushed underground. Sex workers are diverse. While most are female, there are male and transgendered sex workers as well, from young to old. Sex workers often have significantly higher rates of HIV infection than the general population, and preventing transmission among those with multiple sex partners is cost effective in stemming the transmission of HIV to the general population. In addition, according to UNAIDS, "sex workers are among the most likely to respond positively to prevention programmes."

While some adult women and men may enter sex work freely as an occupational choice, many are compelled by coercion or economic circumstances. Violence, trafficking, and debt bondage may be used to coerce people into sex work. Many adults entered sex work as children (see Topic 8.3). Dire economic circumstances also force many into sex work, as it may be the only means of subsistence, or the best-paying option. Sex work may be informal or formal. Informal sex work consists of individual prostitution, including streetwalkers and call-girls or boys, who usually find their clients independently. Many of these sex workers may work sporadically when funds are needed, and not consider themselves to be sex workers. Formal, or organized prostitution employs intermediaries (pimps) between the sex worker and client. Formal prostitution is often centered in brothels, night-clubs, and massage parlors.

Sex workers are especially vulnerable to HIV because stigmatization and discrimination may cause them to avoid health care and pursuing legal remedies against violence. There are seldom laws protecting sex workers, and when there are such laws, they often are not enforced. Limited information on health and risk of HIV infection, as well as limited power to negotiate safer sex place sex workers further at risk. If sex workers use intravenous drugs, alcohol, or have other sexually transmitted infections, their risk of HIV infection is increased.

Legal and Policy Considerations

Sex work is typically treated in one of three ways by a government. Direct prohibition of sex work involves laws criminalizing activities related to commercial sex—solicitation, exchange of sex for money, management of sex workers (pimping or brothel-keeping), and procurement. Alternatively, sex work may be allowed and regulated. States may regulate sex work, including licensing and registering sex workers, brothel owners and/or pimps, mandatory health screenings, and sanitation and/or safe sex requirements. A nation may also have an absence of any regulation regarding prostitution. Decriminalization refers to the movement to normalize or legalize sex work; proponents support a wide range of regulatory frameworks, from minimal state interference, to strong health regulations and protections for the right to association.

Criminalization of sex work and solicitation of sex is the norm in many developing countries, across the Middle East, and in most of the United States. In some countries, such as Australia (partially decriminalized or licensed in most states, fully decriminalized in the state of New South Wales), Brazil, Greece, Kenya, and Bangladesh, sex work is legal and sex workers are entitled to the same rights and benefits as other workers, at least under the law. In practice, however, they may be subjected to discrimination in the legal system (see Topic 5.2). In countries where there is an absence of legal regulation (for example, in Azerbaijan, Bulgaria, Poland, and Slovenia), sex work is not regulated, but sex workers may find themselves prosecuted under a variety of alternative statutes (see Topic 5.2). In countries where individual prostitution is legal or not explicitly illegal, formal prostitution is generally illegal (pimping and brothel-keeping).

The criminalization of sex work may make reaching sex working populations with public health interventions difficult. Government organizations or aid agencies will have difficulty locating and staying in touch with target populations. Fear of prosecution, stigmatization, and discrimination also will keep sex workers from accessing appropriate health care. These circumstances exacerbate the susceptibility of sex workers to becoming infected with HIV and may undermine education and prevention efforts that would reduce HIV transmission among sex workers and their clients.

In places where sex work is unlawful, those engaged in the practice may not avail themselves of legal protection against rape and violence. Even if they do seek redress through the legal system, they are unlikely to be successful due to stigmatization and discrimination. These circumstances make sex workers more vulnerable to violence and to HIV infection.

Practice Examples

In Russia, individual prostitution and pimping are administrative offences subject to a fine; pimping may also be punishable by short-term imprisonment. Brothel-keeping is a criminal offence, punishable by up to three years imprisonment. This is typical of many countries, where individual sex work is generally a low-level offense with more organized forms being subjected to greater penalties.

In Latvia, individual sex work is permitted, subject to a regulatory regime that includes the issuance of a "health card." Regulatory regimes that apply to sex work are discussed further in Topic 5.4.

Azerbaijan, Bulgaria, Kazakhstan, and Poland are examples of countries where there is an absence of legal regulation of sex work.

In 2003, New Zealand decriminalized prostitution in its *Prostitution Reform Act.* The Act permits and regulates sex work, but prohibits sex work by those younger than 18 years of age. The Act requires that all reasonable steps be taken to use an appropriate barrier (condom) if the act engaged in is likely to transmit infection. (http://www.legislation.govt.nz/libraries/contents/om_isapi .dll?clientID =92088&infobase=pal_statutes.nfo&jump=a2003-028&softpage=DOC)

Given the legalized status of sex work, the New Zealand Department of Labour published information useful to protecting the health of sex workers: *A Guide to Occupational Health and Safety in the New Zealand Sex Industry.*

References

Canadian HIV/AIDS Legal Network, *Sex, Work, Rights: Reforming Canadian Criminal Laws on Prostitution* (Canadian HIV/AIDS Legal Network 2005). http://www.aidslaw.ca/ publications/publicationsdocEN.php?ref=199

Central and Eastern European Harm Reduction Network, *Sex Work, HIV/AIDS, and Human Rights in Central and Eastern Europe and Central Asia* (Open Society Institute 2005).

Lawyers Collective, *Legislating an Epidemic: HIV/AIDS in India,* Chapter 8 (Universal Law Publishing Co. Pvt. Ltd. 2005).

Malek, Danielle, *Australia's Successful Response to AIDS and the Role of Law Reform* (Global HIV/AIDS Program, World Bank 2006).

New Zealand Department of Labor, *A Guide to Occupational Health and Safety in the New Zealand Sex Industry* (Department of Labor 2004). http://www.osh.govt.nz/order/ catalogue/pdf/sexindustry.pdf

Pekart, Michael L., *Sex-Work Harm Reduction,* 366 Lancet 2123 (2005).

UNAIDS, *Sex Work and HIV/AIDS: Technical Update* (UNAIDS 2002). http://data.unaids.org/ Publications/IRC-pub02/JC705-SexWork-TU_en.pdf

UNFPA, *HIV/AIDS, Gender, and Sex Work,* Fact Sheet (United Nations Population Fund 2002).

5.2 Vague Criminal Statutes and Police Harassment

The Issue

Regardless of the official legal status of sex work, police and other government officials often interfere with the rights of sex workers. Instead of using criminal statutes against prostitution, the police may target sex workers using various other laws. Police may harass sex workers based on vague statutes on loitering, vagrancy, breach of public order, or hooliganism (among others), or for the lack of appropriate documentation (passport, residency permit, etc.). These actions often contribute to the marginalization of sex workers, which in turn heightens the possibility that they will become infected with HIV.

Legal and Policy Considerations

Legislators, policy makers, the courts, and the police have a role to play in ensuring that laws are not overbroad, vague, or arbitrarily or discriminatorily enforced. Regardless of the legal status of sex work, sex workers must have access to the legal system to protect themselves against rape and violence. The police must be allies in public health and safety. Proper training and enforcement and oversight mechanisms can ensure that this is the case.

There may be little or no relationship between the legal regulations regarding sex work and the practices of police in some regions. Even where individual sex work is legal, police may arrest or detain sex workers on the basis of alternative legal provisions. Police may also use their power or the threat of arrest to extort bribes or sexual favors. Vague laws, such as those that aim to prohibit loitering or breach of public order, are open to interpretation and exploitation by police. Such vague laws offend important tenets of the rule of law. Clear laws give people a reasonable opportunity to know what is permitted and what is proscribed. Vague laws do not provide fair warning, and may trap the innocent. In addition, vague laws provide room for curbside determinations of what is permitted, allowing arbitrary and discriminatory enforcement. By promulgating vague laws, policy makers delegate basic policy decisions to police officers and the courts on an ad hoc basis, undermining the clarity and predictability of the law. Because vague laws open the door to arbitrary and discriminatory application, legislators and policy makers should take care to avoid undue vagueness.

In addition to using tangentially-related or vague laws to persecute sex workers, police in some areas go outside of the law and take advantage of their positions of power. Group rape sessions of sex workers have been reported in police line-ups. Sex workers report having to bribe police officers or provide free sex. Police have beaten sex workers even when they were engaged in lawful, nonsex industry related activities, such as waiting for a bus. Police may refuse to take the complaints of sex workers, may beat them while in custody, and may refuse to present arrested sex workers to a magistrate or judge in violation of due process. Aid workers and peer educators have also been targeted by police. At times, police action directly conflicts with national policies. For example, where government programs financially support aid agencies and the distribution of condoms, local police may sabotage health protection by arresting aid workers or those found in possession of condoms.

Police harassment has severe negative health consequences for sex workers. First, there is the damage done by the police themselves through rape and other forms of physical violence. Verbal abuse by police adds to the negative psychological consequences of sex work. The indirect effects are also important. Sex workers harassed by police are likely to go further underground, outside of the reach of public health officials and aid workers, and therefore more susceptible to HIV infection. Such workers will have limited access to information regarding safe health practices and limited means to protect themselves, leading to increased violence and its negative health effects. Without access to information and condoms, they may transmit HIV to their clients who may transmit it to their other sexual partners.

Proper training of police and local officials can reduce the amount of abuse. Sensitivity training may alert police to the necessity of policies that honor the dignity of sex workers and ensure that aid is not disrupted. In addition, clear laws that limit the opportunity for arbitrary and discriminatory practices are essential, as is the enforcement of laws against police officers who commit violence against sex workers.

Practice Example

In *Johnson v. Carson,* a United States court struck down a statute that prohibited loitering for the purpose of soliciting prostitution. The court found the statute to be vague, because under the wording of the statute, a person could be arrested for innocent activities such as standing on a street and talking to passers-by. Under the statute, known prostitutes could be arrested for waiting for a bus or standing in any public place. (569 F. Supp. 974 M.D. Fla. 1983)

References

Berg, Joel D., *The Troubled Constitutionality of Antigang Loitering Laws,* 69 Chi.-Kent L. Rev. 461 (1993).

Burris, Scott & Daniel Villena, *Adapting to the Reality of HIV: Difficult Policy Choices in Russia, China and India,* 31 Human Rights Magazine 10 (2004).

Human Rights Watch, *Epidemic of Abuse: Police Harassment of HIV/AIDS Outreach Workers in India* (Human Rights Watch 2002). http://www.hrw.org/reports/2002/india2/index.htm#TopOfPage

Lawyers Collective, *Legislating an Epidemic: HIV/AIDS in India,* Chapter 8 (Universal Law Publishing Co. Pvt. Ltd. 2005).

Pekart, Michael L., *Sex-Work Harm Reduction,* 366 Lancet 2123 (2005).

UNAIDS, *Sex Work and HIV/AIDS: Technical Update* (UNAIDS 2002). http://data.unaids.org/Publications/IRC-pub02/JC705-SexWork-TU_en.pdf

5.3 Regulatory Regimes (Labor, Health, Occupational Safety)

The Issue

While many countries criminalize sex workers under the law and subject them to harassment and vilification, some jurisdictions have chosen instead to decriminalize, normalize, and regulate sex work. The UNAIDS & IPU *Handbook for Legislators on HIV/AIDS, Law, and Human Rights* recommends this approach, endorsing decriminalization of sex work where no victimization is involved, and regulation through occupational health and safety standards. These standards can create a less judgmental framework within which public health efforts are more likely to succeed. In turn, decriminalization and regulation can help to protect sex workers as well as their clients from dangers including HIV transmission and violence.

Legal and Policy Considerations

Regulatory regimes that have been applied to sex workers include regulations specific to the sex industry as well as those generally applicable to occupational health and safety regimes. Some of the rules common to the regulation of sex workers are designed to limit the transmission of sexually transmitted diseases and otherwise protect sex workers from danger and violence in the workplace. Common features of regulation include establishing "tolerance zones," or areas of a town, city, or state where sex work is permissible. Inside these tolerance zones, sex workers should not be subjected to harassment or detention by the police.

Many regulations also require periodic (ranging from every week to every three months or less frequent) testing for sexually transmitted infections. These provisions often include an identification, work permit card, or certification that is given only if test results are negative (or, alternatively, the document notes that a test result was positive). Regulations may also require that these cards be registered with the police. When considering any sex-industry specific regulations, it is important to consider that controls on operators or workers that are extremely onerous may spark a second, illegal industry, where no regulations are enforced and health education does not penetrate.

More helpful regulation includes requiring safe sex, as well as the provision of condoms by establishments. Posting notices regarding the requirement of the use of a condom in multiple languages ensures that both clients and sex workers are aware of their obligations. (The success of Thailand's 100% condom rule in sex work is discussed in Topic 5.5.) Regulations or codes of practice may also cover the storage and handling of condoms, sex toys, and other equipment to ensure safety. Consistent use of prophylactics and hygienic practices contribute to HIV prevention strategies and minimize the risk of HIV transmission.

Violence in the workplace is more prevalent in sex work than in other industries, as may be the use of alcohol or drugs. Employee training regarding the effective use of personal protection equipment (from condoms to panic buttons) as well as conflict management and substance abuse awareness can improve the safety of sex workers, decrease violence, and decrease transmission of HIV.

In addition to regulations applying only to the sex industry, the occupational health and safety regulations of a country can be made applicable to sex work when such industries are decriminalized. Sex workers who work through brothels are often considered by the managers to be independent contractors. Regulations that force such workers to be considered employees may afford them protections such as holiday and sick leave, vacation time and workers' compensation, as well as more effectively impose the obligation to pay taxes. These protections may help in ensuring the good health of sex workers, as they would be able to take time off when ill and may qualify for health insurance or services. As the presence of other sexually transmitted infections may increase the likelihood of transmission of HIV, healthy sex workers would be more resistant to HIV should they be exposed. Occupational safety regulations generally require the employer to maintain a safe working environment. In the sex industry, this would include maintaining a clean work environment, providing towels and linens, and minimizing the likelihood of repetitive stress injuries.

In some jurisdictions, other occupational safety standards apply. For example, first aid kits may be required in workplaces, fire safety standards are imposed, and heating, cooling, and lighting requirements exist. Ensuring that workplace safety standards apply to the sex industry creates healthier work environments.

Practice Example

New Zealand's *Prostitution Reform Act of 2003* decriminalized prostitution. (http://www.legislation.govt.nz/libraries/contents/om_isapi.dll?clientID=92088 &infobase=pal_statutes.nfo&jump=a2003-028&softpage=DOC)

A comprehensive guide to occupational health and safety for the New Zealand Sex Industry was developed in conjunction with sex workers' rights organizations. (http://www.osh.govt.nz/order/catalogue/pdf/sexindustry.pdf)

References

Central and Eastern European Harm Reduction Network, *Sex Work, HIV/AIDS, and Human Rights in Central and Eastern Europe and Central Asia* (Open Society Institute 2005). http://www.soros.org/initiatives/health/focus/sharp/articles_publications/publications/ sexwork_20051018/sex%20work%20in%20ceeca_report_2005.pdf

Jones, Kevin, ed., *Safety at Work,* (Workplace Safety Services Pty Ltd 2000). http://www
.walnet.org/csis/safety/SAFEWORK.PDF

UNAIDS, *Sex Work and HIV/AIDS: Technical Update* (UNAIDS 2002). http://data.unaids
.org/Publications/IRC-pub02/JC705-SexWork-TU_en.pdf

UNAIDS & IPU, *Handbook for Legislators on HIV/AIDS, Law and Human Rights: Action to
Combat HIV/AIDS in View of Its Devastating Human, Economic, and Social Impact*
(UNAIDS & Inter-Parliamentary Union 1999). http://www.ipu.org/PDF/publications/
aids_en.pdf

5.4 100% Condom Use Programs

The Issue

In the early years of the HIV pandemic, Thailand's sex industry was a significant source of infection in the country. Though sex work has been illegal in Thailand since 1960, in practice the government has adopted harm reduction strategies to control rather than eradicate it. In 1989, the "100% condom use program" was piloted in Thailand's Ratchaburi province. The program combined free, easily accessible condoms with a requirement that sex workers and clients use condoms for all sexual acts that could result in HIV transmission. Sex workers who sought treatment at government clinics were offered free, unlimited access to condoms, and health officials who visited commercial sex establishments brought condoms with them. A "No Condom—No Sex" policy was implemented, and enforced through sanctions against noncooperative establishments, which could be shut down for a period of time or closed permanently. This policy gave establishment managers the incentive to support sex workers in negotiating condom use. Men seeking treatment for sexually transmitted infections at government clinics would be asked if they had visited a commercial sex establishment, and whether or not condoms were used. (Contact tracing was an already-established part of sexually transmitted infection control in Thailand.) In this way, establishments not enforcing the 100% condom use program were discovered. Because most establishments then required condom use, there was a decrease in market pressure for condom-free sex.

After success in Ratchaburi, in 1991, the program was implemented nationally with the endorsement of the Prime Minister, and it has been successful in damp- ening the transmission of HIV. By 2000, 96% of sex workers used condoms and Thailand saw a 90% reduction in sexually transmitted infections among men treated at government clinics. However, in recent years, government support for the program may have flagged. Messages about condom use appear to be less prevalent, as is funding for condoms. Fewer people are reached by the program, and some may falsely assume that with the messages about AIDS disappearing, the disease is no longer a threat.

Legal and Policy Considerations

The WHO identifies six strategies essential to a successful 100% condom use program (CUP). The first is high-level political commitment. Even where prosti- tution is illegal, a CUP can be implemented, but doing so requires the commit- ment of the political structures. If sex workers are arrested for carrying or buying condoms, the program cannot be implemented. Political commitment can be demonstrated through the appropriate local medium (i.e., by regulation, decree, or proclamation).

Second, institutional structures must be established to manage the program. Community, business, political, and professional leaders; technical staff from governmental agencies; representatives of the sex trade; and NGOs should be convened to design the policy.

Third, the program requires that quality condoms be promoted and accessible. The fourth element works in conjunction with the third: commercial sex establishments must be identified and sought for collaboration in the program.

Fifth, condom use should be monitored to ensure that there is compliance, and sixth, the outcome and impact of the program should be evaluated. CUPs can be monitored as in Thailand, using established facilities that diagnose and treat sexually transmitted infections in males. In other areas, infection information is gathered from sex workers during routine health screenings, or "mystery clients" test actual practice.

While CUPs have been shown to be effective in increasing condom usage in the formal sector, informal/individual sex work is more difficult to monitor. Some critics suggest that CUPs result in sex workers leaving brothel environments, either because they are forced to due to their health status, their brothel is closed by the government policy, or they are drawn to the underground market of condom-free sex. Other critics of these programs claim that CUPs promote sex work or illegal behavior. However, the programs can be seen as taking no stance on the value of sex work or the criminality of the activity, but focusing on the public health aspects of the reality of sex work. Other critics claim that the system is vulnerable to bribery, or does not acknowledge the rights of sex workers who may be forced to engage in the work and need more systemic government intervention.

Practice Examples

In addition to Thailand, several other countries have implemented a CUP. These include Cambodia, the Dominican Republic, Vietnam, China, Myanmar, and the Philippines, among others.

References

BBC, *Chinks in Thailand's AIDS Armour,* BBC News (Dec. 1, 2000). http://news.bbc.co.uk/1/hi/world/asia-pacific/1049794.stm

Hanenberg, Robert & Wiwat Rojanapithayakorn, *Prevention as Policy: How Thailand Reduced STD and HIV Transmission,* 3 AIDSCaption (1996).

Network of Sex Work Projects, *The 100% Condom Use Policy: A Sex Worker Rights Perspective* (Network of Sex Work Projects 2003). http://www.nswp.org/safety/100percent.html

UNAIDS, *Evaluation of the 100% Condom Programme in Thailand: Case Study* (UNAIDS 2000). http://data.unaids.org/Publications/IRC-pub01/JC275-100pCondom_en.pdf

WHO, *Experiences of 100% Condom Use Programme in Selected Countries of Asia* (World Health Organization 2004). http://www.wpro.who.int/publications/pub_9290610921.htm

———, *Responding to Questions about the 100% Condom Use Programme: An Aid for Programme Staff* (World Health Organization 2004). http://www.wpro.who.int/publications/pub_9290610867.htm

———, *Thailand Achieves Sustained Reduction in HIV Infection Rates,* in Health, A Key to Prosperity, Success Stories in Developing Countries (World Health Organization 2000). http://www.who.int/inf-new/aids1.htm

5.5 Trafficking of Women for Sex Work

The Issue

Trafficking in persons, in addition to being a grave violation of human rights, fuels the spread of HIV. Like noncoercive forms of migration, trafficking poses the possibility of transmitting infections from one geographic location to another. However, unlike traditional immigration, those who have been trafficked are less likely to seek help or medical treatment due to fear of being exposed as a prostitute, of violence and debt, and of being in the country illegally. In addition to language and cultural barriers, and a lack of information about legal rights, these factors make reaching trafficked people with rescue and/or public health messages difficult.

Legal and Policy Considerations

Trafficking is defined in the United Nations *Protocol to Prevent, Suppress and Punish Trafficking in Persons, especially Women and Children* as "the recruitment, transportation, transfer, harbouring or receipt of persons, by means of the threat or use of force or other forms of coercion, of abduction, of fraud, of deception, of the abuse of power or of a position of vulnerability or of the giving or receiving of payments or benefits to achieve the consent of a person having control over another person, for the purpose of exploitation. Exploitation shall include, at a minimum, the exploitation of the prostitution of others or other forms of sexual exploitation, forced labour or services, slavery, servitude or the removal of organs."

Traditionally, victims of trafficking were seen as criminals and often prosecuted for prostitution or related offenses. While over 150 countries had some law that applied to trafficking, these were rarely invoked. Often, those trafficked went to jail and the traffickers went free. Since the U.N. Protocol was adopted in 2000, laws that correctly identify trafficked people as victims are becoming more prevalent.

Trafficked people are brought across state lines under coercion or false pretenses, and trapped into cooperating with their traffickers. Those trafficked will not come forward for protection or health care if they are afraid of legal prosecution. Treating those trafficked as victims, instead of prosecuting them, has the benefit of increased cooperation with law enforcement officials and therefore the prosecution of those doing the trafficking. Treating trafficked people as lawbreakers undermines their human rights and complicates efforts to protect them from contracting or spreading HIV. They should not be criminally liable for prostitution, illegal entry, falsification of documents, or other related offenses, and some states now prevent such liability under law (see practice example below). Many states also do not require the victims to testify as a prerequisite for the trafficking acts conducted to be considered criminal. Victimized populations may be weary of formal legal institutions, injured, and traumatized, and should not be forced to testify.

Stopping trafficking in human beings requires national law that recognizes trafficking as a serious crime and establishes stiff penalties. For example, under the European Council Framework Decision of July 19, 2002, European countries must provide trafficking penalties of at least eight years imprisonment. Penalties should be enhanced for aggravated circumstances (including trafficking vulnerable persons, such as children).

Victims of trafficking should be made safe. This may include witness protection programs and protection from traffickers. Laws may also provide compensation or restitution to the victims of trafficking, and should require the forfeiture of assets gained by traffickers. Confiscated assets can be used to compensate the victim directly or to provide funding for victim services. Services provided to victims of trafficking may include medical, legal, psychological, and social aid. According to the U.N. protocol, victims may need access to appropriate housing, counseling regarding legal options, medical and psychological treatment, and employment or training opportunities.

Those trafficked should be entitled to seek residency in the destination country. Rapid repatriation of victims can further endanger them, and hinders law enforcement. Some countries, including Belgium, Italy, the Netherlands, and the United States allow temporary or permanent residence for victims of trafficking. Deportation is still the norm in most other parts of the world. Those wishing to return to their country of origin should be able to return with dignity and respect with the assistance of the country of origin.

Practice Examples

In addition to the U.N. Protocol (http://untreaty.un.org/English/notpubl/18-12-a.E.doc), the Council of Europe *Convention on Action against Trafficking in Human Beings* (http://www.coe.int/T/E/human_rights/trafficking/PDF_Conv_197_Trafficking_E.pdf) and the U.S. Office to Monitor and Combat Trafficking in Persons *Model Law to Combat Trafficking in Persons* (http://www.usdoj.gov/crt/crim/model_state_law.pdf) are helpful resources. These documents contain provisions protective of victims of trafficking that can be used to combat the crime and promote health. National laws in the United States, Dominican Republic, Moldova, the Kyrgyz Republic, and Romania do not criminalize trafficking victims.

In Italy, a trafficker's property can be confiscated when its value appears out of all proportions to the owner's legal income. (*Confisca di Beni ai Sensi Dell'art* [Confiscation of Criminal Assets] No. 356, 1992)

References

Lawyers Collective, *Legislating an Epidemic: HIV/AIDS in India*, Chapter 8 (Universal Law Publishing Co. Pvt. Ltd. 2005).

Mattar, Y., *Incorporating the Five Basic Elements of Model Antitrafficking in Persons Legislation in Domestic Laws: From the United Nations Protocol to the European Convention*, 14 Tul. J. Int'l & Comp. L. 357 (2006).

UNAIDS, *Sex Work and HIV/AIDS: Technical Update* (UNAIDS 2002). http://data.unaids.org/Publications/IRC-pub02/JC705-SexWork-TU_en.pdf

UNODC, *Trafficking in Persons: Global Patterns* (United Nations Office on Drugs and Crime 2006). http://www.unodc.org/pdf/traffickinginpersons_report_2006ver2.pdf

United States Office to Monitor and Combat Trafficking in Persons, *Model Law to Combat Trafficking in Persons* (United States Office to Monitor and Combat Trafficking in Persons, accessed 04/13/2007). http://www.usdoj.gov/crt/crim/model_state_law.pdf

SECTION 6

Men Having Sex with Men

6.1 Gender Orientation in General Antidiscrimination Statutes

The Issue

Men who have sex with men (MSM) are at high risk of contracting HIV, but their opportunities for protection from infection may be reduced by societal discrimination. MSM may hide their sexual orientation, fearing discrimination from their community, government, employers, insurers, and others. As a result, they are less likely to seek HIV prevention, diagnosis, and treatment services. Improving protections from discrimination on the basis of sexual orientation may alleviate the need for secrecy and make it easier to reach the MSM population with HIV prevention efforts.

Legal and Policy Considerations

Legal antidiscrimination protections for persons on the basis of their sexual orientation vary internationally in theory and practice. Some countries (e.g., South Africa, Australia, and countries in the EU—see below) provide such protections via constitutional or statutory laws. These laws are consistent with human rights norms. Several international human rights documents, such as the *International Covenant on Civil and Political Rights* (ICCPR), mention or have been interpreted to include antidiscrimination protections based on sexual orientation. The Supreme Court of India has ruled that in the absence of appropriate national legislation, international treaties signed by India (including the ICCPR) have the force of law. In India and other countries with similar rulings, the ICCPR and other human rights documents may thus provide antidiscrimination protections for individuals with respect to gender orientation and their HIV-positive status. Still many countries do not provide substantive legal protections from discrimination based on sexual orientation. As well, human rights norms in many countries may not be applied so as to result in meaningful protections.

Practice Examples

The 1994 case, *Toonen vs. Australia,* led the U.N. Human Rights Committee (now the U.N. Human Rights Council) to conclude that the references to "sex" in Articles 2, paragraph 1, (nondiscrimination) and 26 (equality before the law) of the 1966 International Covenant on Civil and Political Rights (ICCPR) should be interpreted to include sexual orientation:

> *Article 2*—(1) Each State Party to the present Covenant undertakes to respect and to ensure to all individuals within its territory and subject to its jurisdiction the rights recognized in the present Covenant, without

distinction of any kind, such as race, colour, *sex,* language, religion, political or other opinion, national or social origin, property, birth or other status. (Emphasis added.)

Article 26—All persons are equal before the law and are entitled without any discrimination to the equal protection of the law. In this respect, the law shall prohibit any discrimination and guarantee to all persons equal and effective protection against discrimination on any ground such as race, colour, *sex,* language, religion, political or other opinion, national or social origin, property, birth or other status. (Emphasis added.)

Toonen led to the repeal of the prohibition on male same-sex acts in the Tasmanian Criminal Code. Subsequently the Tasmanian Parliament adopted "the most progressive antidiscrimination legislation in Australia." (Malek 2006 cites extracts of the Tasmanian Anti-Discrimination Act 1998 at 11–13.)

On the supranational level, the European Union Council *Directive 2000/78/EC* of 27 November 2000 established a general antidiscrimination framework in employment and occupation, which requires individual national legislation to come into effect in each Member State: (12) "To this end, any direct or indirect discrimination based on religion or belief, disability, age or *sexual orientation* as regards the areas covered by this Directive should be prohibited throughout the Community." (Emphasis added.)

On the national level, South Africa enshrines the protection of individuals from discrimination based on sexual orientation in its 1996 Constitution: 2.9 (3) "The state may not unfairly discriminate directly or indirectly against anyone on one or more grounds, including race, gender, sex, pregnancy, marital status, ethnic or social origin, colour, *sexual orientation,* age, disability, religion, conscience, belief, culture, language and birth." (Emphasis added.) The Constitutional Court of South Africa has enforced this clause in a series of judgments. See Human Rights Watch, Resource Library for International Jurisprudence on Sexual Orientation and Gender Identity.

References

AIDS Law Project & AIDS Legal Network, *HIV/AIDS and the Law: A Resource Manual,* Chapter 10 (3rd ed. AIDS Law Project & AIDS Legal Network 2003).

Human Rights Watch, *Resource Library for International Jurisprudence on Sexual Orientation and Gender Identity* (Human Rights Watch, accessed 04/13/2007). http://hrw.org/lgbt/jurisprudence.htm#3

IGLHRC, *International Jurisprudence and Policy Precedents Regarding Sexual Orientation* (International Gay and Lesbian Human Rights Commission 1996). http://www.iglhrc.org/files/iglhrc/reports/990430-intljuris.pdf

ILGA, *Anti-Discrimination and Anti-Vilification Legislation* (International Lesbian and Gay Association, accessed 04/13/2007). http://www.ilga.info/Information/Legal_survey/ Subject_specific_resources_&_useful_documents.htm

Lawyers' Collective, *Legislating an Epidemic: HIV/AIDS in India*, Chapter 6 (Universal Law Publishing Co. Pvt. Ltd. 2003).

Malek, Danielle, *Australia's Successful Response to AIDS and the Role of Law Reform* (Global HIV/AIDS Program, World Bank 2006).

Responsibilities: Male Sexual Health and HIV in Asia and the Pacific International Consultation, *The Delhi Declaration of Collaboration*, September 23–26, 2006. http:// risksandresponsibilities.org/DelhiDeclaration_Full.pdf

UNAIDS, *AIDS and Men Who Have Sex with Men: UNAIDS Technical Update* (UNAIDS 2000). http://data.unaids.org/Publications/IRC-pub03/mentu2000_en.pdf

———, *HIV and Sex between Men: UNAIDS Policy Brief* (UNAIDS 2006). http://data .unaids.org/pub/BriefingNote/2006/20060801_Policy_Brief_MSM_en.pdf

UNHRC, *Toonen v. Australia*, UN Doc. CCPR/C/50/D/488/1992, decision of March 31 (United Nations Human Rights Council 1994). http://hrw.org/lgbt/pdf/toonen.pdf

Wikipedia, *Homosexuality Laws of the World* (Wikipedia, accessed 04/13/2007). http://en .wikipedia.org/wiki/Homosexuality_laws_of_the_world

6.2   Sexual Offenses

The Issue

MSM have often been discriminated against through statutes (and other laws) that criminalize consensual homosexual acts. In addition, MSM have at times become the targets of unwanted sexual attacks. In certain situations, they may find themselves victims of rape, especially among subgroups of male sex workers and prison populations. In men-only penal institutions, homosexual acts can contribute to higher HIV prevalence. Specific protective measures may prevent the spread of HIV for MSM. However, secrecy surrounding homosexual acts and governments' failure to address them because of the stigma associated with MSM increase HIV risk. Social stigma gives rise to laws prohibiting certain homosexual behaviors. This, in turn, leads to the marginalization of MSM, making them more vulnerable to HIV and AIDS.

Legal and Policy Considerations

Numerous countries have statutes that penalize certain sexual acts between consenting adults, regardless of gender. Often grouped under the term "sodomy laws," they may prohibit specific acts (e.g., anal sex, oral sex) as well as regulate a range of same-sex activity. Many countries actively employ these laws in a discriminatory fashion against MSM. Authorities may selectively enforce these laws against MSM, target MSM for prosecution, or use these offenses as guises for further discrimination.

Some countries, however, have sought to repeal these statutes or limit their discriminatory application. For example, many states in the United States have repealed their sodomy laws following the 2003 United States Supreme Court decision, *Lawrence v. Texas,* which invalidated Texas' antihomosexual laws (and similar laws in other states). In other parts of the world, sexual offense laws targeted at homosexual men vary in degrees of severity of punishments, including fines, corporal abuse, and long-term incarceration. Laws in Iran, Nigeria, Pakistan, Saudi Arabia, and Sudan may impose the death penalty for sexual offenses committed by MSM.

Practice Examples

In *Lawrence v. Texas,* noted above, the U.S. Supreme Court invalidated a Texas sodomy law that made it a crime for two persons of the same sex to engage in "deviate sexual intercourse" (e.g., oral or anal sex). The Court addressed whether liberty interests under the Fourteenth Amendment of the U.S. Constitution protected adults in deciding how to conduct their private lives pertaining to sex. It also addressed whether the government's interest in circumscribing personal choice and criminalizing such behavior outweighed individual liberty interests. The Court reasoned that the Constitution protected the rights of consenting adults to engage in private sexual behavior without government intervention. Criminalizing such conduct not only affronts personal freedoms, it does not further any legitimate state interests so as to justify an intrusion into private lives. The *Lawrence* opinion and corresponding statutory changes recognize the rights of MSM and others to engage in private sexual behaviors without discrimination or other governmental intrusions.

In Singapore, sodomy laws remain and are actively used to discriminate against homosexuals. Besides general statutes against "molestation" and "indecent behavior," the Singapore penal code contains the following articles:

Section 377 (Unnatural Offences): "Whoever voluntarily has carnal intercourse against the order of nature with any man, woman or animal, shall be punished with imprisonment for life, or with imprisonment for a term which may extend to ten years, and shall also be liable to fine."

Section 377A (Outrages on Decency): "Any male person who, in public or private, commits, or abets the commission by any male person, of any act of gross indecency with another male person, shall be punished with imprisonment for a term which may extend to two years."

References

IGLHRC, *Where Having Sex Is a Crime: Criminalization and Decriminalization of Homosexual Acts* (International Gay and Lesbian Human Rights Commission 2003). http://www.iglhrc.org/site/iglhrc/content.php?type=1&id=77

ILGA (International Lesbian and Gay Association). www.ilga.org

Responsibilities: Male Sexual Health and HIV in Asia and the Pacific International Consultation, *The Delhi Declaration of Collaboration,* September 23–26, 2006. http://risksandresponsibilities.org/DelhiDeclaration_Full.pdf

UNAIDS, *Men Who Have Sex with Men* (UNAIDS, accessed 04/13/2007). http://www.unaids.org/en/Issues/Affected_communities/men_who_have_sex_with_men.asp

————, *HIV and Sex between Men: UNAIDS Policy Brief* (UNAIDS 2006). http://data.unaids.org/pub/BriefingNote/2006/20060801_Policy_Brief_MSM_en.pdf

Wikipedia, *Sodomy Law* (Wikipedia, accessed 04/13/2007). http://en.wikipedia.org/wiki/Sodomy_law

Wikipedia, *Sodomy Laws* (Wikipedia, accessed 04/13/2007). http://www.sodomylaws.org/world/singapore/singapore.htm

6.3 Vague or Overbroad Criminal Statutes and Police Harassment

The Issue

Vague criminal statutes are often enacted and enforced in some countries to enable discrimination based on sexual orientation. Police may target certain groups of MSM and arrest them to dissuade them from gathering or meeting in certain areas. Their authority to do so is based in part on over-broad laws that significantly challenge due process norms found in constitutional and human rights provisions. Statutes intended to facilitate the suppression of activities of MSM may also be applied to inhibit the work of intervening agents. Efforts aimed at disseminating information on HIV prevention and safer sex may be hampered by the actions of police acting on the implicit power granted by vague laws. Ultimately, the enforcement of these criminal statutes leads to public humiliations and infringements of rights of MSM.

Legal and Policy Considerations

MSM are often targeted for prosecution or harassment through laws that are enacted on the grounds of needing to protect the morality and decency of society. These statutes may take the form of laws against "anti-social behavior," "immoral behavior," "causing a public scandal," or "loitering," among others. Police may use these laws to arrest people known to be or suspected of being MSM. Agents of NGOs that try to help MSM can be targeted through the same statutes or may be charged for abetment of a criminal offense. Laws that prohibit "promotion of homosexuality" have been used to prevent distribution of materials dealing with safer sex and public health issues faced by MSM.

In addition to public harassment, police authorities in certain countries have been known to go beyond disbanding gatherings of MSM to include arrest and abuse. In a 2002 survey conducted in Senegal, thirteen percent of MSM reported being raped by a policeman who used the imprimatur of his authority to coerce victims. A study on rights abuses in Kazakhstan revealed that male and transgender sex workers are regularly raped, beaten, and subject to extortion by the police. In these and other examples, police may use laws that discourage homosexual behavior to justify their discrimination (see the example of Jamaica, below) or other offensive acts.

Numerous international documents seek to protect the rights of MSM against these abuses and allow dissemination of public health and HIV materials aimed at this population, as well as other protective tools, such as condoms. Pursuant to international human rights norms (e.g., the right of individuals to the highest attainable standard of health), states must not withhold or prevent the sharing of HIV (or other) health information with populations on any discriminatory basis, including sexual orientation. However, on a practical level, some countries may apply their laws in an over-broad manner to discriminate against MSM.

Practice Example

Jamaica's *Offenses against the Person Act* provides an example of the broad range of powers possessed by the police that may lead to discrimination against MSM. Section 80 of the Act allows the police to arrest without a warrant any person found "loitering in any highway, yard or other place" between 7 p.m. and 6 a.m. if the police officer has "good cause to suspect" that the person had committed or is about to commit a felony. In addition, Section 3(r) and Section 4 of the *Towns and Communities Act* of Jamaica vest police with the power to arrest a person without a warrant based on charges made by a "credible person" that a certain offense has been committed. According to Human Rights Watch, these laws are often applied to MSM. MSM may also be charged with "buggary" (the definition of which includes anal sex), a felony that carries a maximum punishment of ten years including hard labor. Frequently, Jamaica's vague statutes are also used to inhibit HIV/AIDS workers from handing out condoms or disseminating information. Due to legal restrictions, the Jamaican Ministry of Health will not promote services aimed at helping MSM. Rather, it leaves the task to Jamaica AIDS Support, an NGO whose workers may face harassment and abuse by law enforcement officials and the community.

References

Human Rights Watch, *Hated to Death: Homophobia, Violence and Jamaica's HIV/AIDS Epidemic,* 16(6B) Human Rights Watch (2004). http://hrw.org/reports/2004/jamaica1104/jamaica1104.pdf

ILGA (International Lesbian and Gay Association). http://www.ilga.org

Institute of Environmental Sciences, *Meeting the Sexual Health Needs of Men Who Have Sex with Men in Senegal* (Cheikh Anta Diop University, Senegal National AIDS Control Council, Horizons Program 2002).

Responsibilities: Male Sexual Health and HIV in Asia and the Pacific International Consultation, *The Delhi Declaration of Collaboration*, September 23–26, 2006. http://risksandresponsibilities.org/DelhiDeclaration_Full.pdf

UNAIDS, *HIV and Sex between Men: UNAIDS Policy Brief* (UNAIDS 2006). http://data.unaids.org/pub/BriefingNote/2006/20060801_Policy_Brief_MSM_en.pdf

UNAIDS, UNICEF & WHO (World Health Organization), *Breaking the Barriers: Partnership to Fight HIV/AIDS in Europe and Central Asia* (Ministerial Conference, Dublin, February 23–24, 2004).

6.4 Rights of Association and Expression

The Issue

The rights to association and expression have been recognized as basic legal and human rights to which everyone is entitled in many national and regional constitutions. For persons with HIV, these freedoms may further their access to prevention and treatment, and assure them opportunities to congregate to express their concerns and needs. However, because of the social stigma attached to MSM, their rights can be curtailed through laws (e.g., against the promotion of homosexuality) as well as their own self-restrictions. MSM may be discouraged from meeting in public places, expressing their opinions and creative endeavors, participating in public health programs or research, and seeking public health services. Consequently they may be driven deeper underground making HIV prevention efforts less effectual.

Legal and Policy Considerations

The *Universal Declaration of Human Rights* (UDHR) protects the right to freedom of expression in Article 19, which states that: "everyone has the right to freedom of opinion and expression; this right includes freedom to hold opinions without interference and to seek, receive and impart information and ideas through any media and regardless of frontiers." Similarly, Article 20 protects the right to "freedom of peaceful assembly and association." The *International Covenant on Civil and Political Rights* (ICCPR) also protects the right to freedom of expression (Article 19) and the rights to peaceful assembly (Article 21) and association with others (Article 22).

On a national level, laws vary from country to country in the degree of freedoms that they allow MSM (and others) in exercising their rights to association and expression. In some countries, such as Saudi Arabia, the law does not guarantee the rights to association or expression to its citizens. Other countries may place implicit or explicit restrictions on the rights of expression and association. For example, they may make the rights contingent on the preservation of "public order" or "morality" (see example of Honduras, below). Although a country's laws may guarantee rights to association and expression seemingly without restriction, in practice, these rights of MSM are dependent on the extent to which the laws are respected and enforced as well as the extent to which society is educated on and open to gender orientation issues.

Practice Examples

The right to expression can be restricted through laws against the "promotion of homosexuality." In the United Kingdom, Section 28 of the *Local Government Act*

1988 states: "[I]t is illegal for local authorities to "intentionally promote homosexuality," publish material with the "intention of promoting homosexuality," or to promote the teaching in schools of "the acceptability of homosexuality as a pretended family relationship."

This law has led to self-censorship by local authorities in providing funding or support for homosexual organizations. In addition, it has been used to justify discrimination and misinterpreted to restrict discussion of topics dealing with homosexuality. The rights of MSM to express themselves are thus curtailed through laws that are vague and seek to uphold a certain vision of societal morality.

The right of MSM to association can also be limited through restrictions on the right to expression. In Honduras, the right to associate may be exercised according to Article 78 of the Constitution so long as it is not "contrary to public order and good morals." According to Amnesty International, in 2004 the Lesbian, Gay, Bisexual and Transgender (LGBT) organization *Grupo Prisma* asked the Ministry of the Interior and Justice for official registration, as required by law. The group outlined in its statutes its objectives, which included bringing together the LGBT community to increase awareness and self-esteem. The Head of the Department of Legal Services denied the application, citing as the reason the belief that the group's Statutes go against "public order and good morals."

References

Amnesty International, *Honduras: The Right to Freedom of Association and LGBT Organizations* (Amnesty International 2004). www.amnesty.org

Human Rights Education Associates, *Study Guide: Sexual Orientation and Human Rights* (Human Rights Education Associates 2003). http://www.hrea.org/learn/guides/lgbt.html# instruments

ILGA, *World Legal Survey* (International Lesbian and Gay Association, accessed 04/13/2007). http://www.ilga.info/Information/Legal_survey/summary_information_by_subject.htm#* Denial

OHCHR, *Introduction to HIV/AIDS and Human Rights* (Office of the United Nations High Commissioner for Human Rights, accessed 04/13/2007). http://www.ohchr.org/english/ issues/hiv/introhiv.htm

Responsibilities: Male Sexual Health and HIV in Asia and the Pacific International Consultation, *The Delhi Declaration of Collaboration,* September 23–26, 2006. http:// risksandresponsibilities.org/DelhiDeclaration_Full.pdf

UNAIDS, *HIV and Sex between Men: UNAIDS Policy Brief* (UNAIDS 2006). http://data .unaids.org/pub/BriefingNote/2006/20060801_Policy_Brief_MSM_en.pdf

SECTION 7

Women

7.1 Access to Medical Treatment

The Issue

Women living with HIV may be routinely subjected to social barriers that decrease their ability to access treatment. Economic factors play a significant role, as women are more likely than men to lack money to pay for medication or transportation to treatment facilities. Women also traditionally assume greater domestic responsibilities, reducing their ability to travel to receive health care. These factors may be exacerbated by gender-based stigma and discrimination directed toward women living with HIV. For example, families with limited resources and multiple HIV-positive members may pay for treatment for the men only. Furthermore, because women may face persecution and violence if their HIV status is revealed, many refuse to seek testing or treatment. However, it should be noted that WHO/UNAIDS data indicate that women's access to treatment is similar to their share of total infections in many countries.

Legal and Policy Considerations

Gender-based disparities in treatment access raise difficult questions about the most effective way to change underlying social norms that negatively impact women. Prohibiting or criminalizing discriminatory behavior is one option to address these disparities. UNAIDS and OHCHR have urged countries to enact antidiscrimination laws that prohibit gender-based discrimination and reduce the vulnerability of women to HIV infection and the impact of HIV and AIDS. Most countries with rising HIV prevalence have laws against sexual violence and rape (see Topics 7.3, 7.5), and some have adopted more progressive property inheritance laws (see Topic 7.2). However, inadequate enforcement undermines the impact of these laws and leaves many HIV-infected women fearful of disclosing their status or seeking treatment. Other inequalities are less susceptible to punitive redress: if a family with limited resources chooses to treat male rather than female members, criminal sanctions are not an appropriate legal response.

These realities call for comprehensive strategies that build governments' capacity to enforce effective laws and create incentives to modify discriminatory practices. To break the economic dependency that puts them at risk, women and girls need greater access to education, income-generating programs, and job training opportunities. Governments can encourage microfinance programs, which have proved successful in empowering and, in some cases, providing specific services for women living with HIV. Governments can also reduce the stigma associated with HIV by integrating testing and treatment with other reproductive health services (e.g., family planning and pre-natal care) that women are more likely to access (see Topic 7.4).

It is important to note that differential access to treatment is not solely a problem in the developing world. In the United States, women have traditionally faced additional barriers to entry into clinical trials for novel HIV therapies. Due to ethical concerns regarding potential harm to the developing fetus, women of childbearing age have been routinely excluded from studies of experimental medications for HIV. Although such therapies are, by definition, unproven, they may represent the only options for women who are ineligible for conventional treatment.

Practice Examples

In 2002, the Constitutional Court of South Africa, the country's highest court, ruled that government restrictions on the availability of nevirapine (an antiretroviral drug proven to be effective and economical in reducing mother-to-child-transmission (MTCT) of HIV) violated the health care rights of women and newborns under the South African constitution. Pregnant women with HIV can now access nevirapine at almost every hospital, health center, and clinic in the country. In addition to reducing MTCT dramatically, this ruling may also increase the likelihood that HIV-positive women will access treatment for their own illness. (*Minister of Health and Others v. Treatment Action Campaign and Others,* CCT 8/02, 2002. http://www.constitutionalcourt.org.za/uhtbin/cgisirsi/qk7wrJLTSp/259850005/9)

The HIV Law Project, a New Yorkbased nonprofit organization, filed a citizens' petition against the US Food and Drug Administration (FDA), calling on the FDA to relax restrictions that prevented many women of childbearing age from participating in clinical trials. The FDA subsequently adopted regulations establishing an optional "clinical hold"—essentially an administrative penalty preventing the study from continuing—on any drug trial to treat a life-threatening illness that excludes women of childbearing age. (21 C.F.R. 312. http://frwebgate.access.gpo.gov/cgibin/getdoc.cgi?dbname=2000_register &docid=00-13664-filed)

References

Albertyn, C., *Using Rights and the Law to Reduce Women's Vulnerability to HIV/AIDS: A Discussion Paper* (Canadian HIV/AIDS Legal Network 2000). www.aidslaw.ca/women

Fleischman, J., *Breaking the Cycle: Ensuring Equitable Access to HIV Treatment for Women and Girls* (Center for Strategic and International Studies 2004). http://www.csis.org/index.php?option=com_csis_pubs&task=view&id=2631

OHCHR, *Convention on the Elimination of All Forms of Discrimination against Women,* Art. 12 (Office of the United Nations High Commissioner for Human Rights 1979). http://www.ohchr.org

UNAIDS, UNFPA & UNIFEM, *Women and HIV/AIDS: Confronting the Crisis* (UNAIDS, United Nations Population Fund & United Nations Development Fund for Women 2004). http://womenandaids.unaids.org/publications.html

WHO & UNAIDS, *Ensuring Equitable Access to Antiretroviral Treatment for Women* (World Health Organization & UNAIDS 2004). http://www.who.int/gender/hiv_aids/en/

——, *Progress on Global Access to HIV Antiretroviral Therapy. A Report on "3 by 5" and Beyond* (World Health Organization & UNAIDS 2006).

7.2   Property Ownership and Inheritance

The Issue

In many developing countries, statutory and customary laws prevent women from owning, controlling, or inheriting property. Upon dissolution of a marriage or death of a spouse, women often lose control over all significant assets. Such exclusion from full property rights carries particularly harmful consequences for divorced or widowed women with HIV, who may be forced into unsanitary living conditions or may no longer be able to afford treatment. Women in this situation may also face difficulties in accessing other basic necessities such as food and shelter, which along with HIV infection can undermine their health even more dramatically. In some circumstances, divorced or widowed women who have no property or job prospects may have to resort to sex work to support themselves, increasing their risk of contracting HIV. If they are infected with HIV, the infection may be passed on to others. For married women, unequal property rights can increase their likelihood of HIV infection by weakening their bargaining position within the relationship, making it more difficult to negotiate safer sex.

Legal and Policy Considerations

International law generally prohibits discrimination against women, including discrimination in marriage and family relations. More specifically, the *Declaration of Commitment on HIV/AIDS* adopted by the U.N. General Assembly in 2001 required governments to enact and enforce legislation to eliminate discrimination in access to inheritance. However, national and local laws and customs do not necessarily reflect a similar commitment to equalizing women's property rights. Legislation explicitly prohibiting women from owning or inheriting land and property has become rare, although many countries lack gender sensitive legislation or a legislative framework that protects women's human rights. The effectiveness of antidiscriminatory inheritance legislation is often limited by numerous exceptions and inadequate enforcement.

In countries where adequate statutory provisions have been enacted to govern land, property, and inheritance, customary law—unwritten social norms that ostensibly reflect community values but which often reinforce gender bias—may still bar women from exercising their rights. In family matters, including the distribution of property after a death, customary law often prevails over more gender-neutral statutory law or states' obligations under international human rights treaties. Some countries' laws explicitly prefer customary law in resolving inheritance disputes, whereas in others the application of customary law reflects a lack of awareness among judges and lawyers about statutory provisions designed to safeguard women's property rights. Enhancing property rights for women will empower them to protect themselves from HIV infection more effectively and allow women living with HIV to access needed care and treatment more successfully.

Practice Examples

In Tanzania, the 1999 *Land Act* and *Village Land Act* include provisions overriding customary laws that restrict women's rights to use, transfer, and own land:

> "Any rule of customary law and any decision taken in respect of land held under customary tenure, whether in respect of land held individually or communally, shall have regard to the custom, traditions, and practices of the community concerned and the rule of customary law or any such decision in respect of land held under customary tenure shall be void and inoperative and shall not be given any effect by any village council or village assembly or any person or body of persons exercising any authority over village land or in respect of any court or other body, to the extent to which it denies women, children or persons with disability lawful access to ownership, occupation or use of any kind." (*Village Land Act, 1999* §20(2))

In addition, the Acts ensure that women are represented in land administration and adjudication bodies. (*Land Act, 1999,* §17; *Village Land Act, 1999,* §§53(2), 53(5), and 60(2))

In a 1996 case, the Supreme Court of India refused to apply a provision of the law that denied women full ownership rights over property acquired by way of gift, will, or other instrument. Citing the Indian Constitution and the *Convention on the Elimination of All Forms of Discrimination against Women* (CEDAW), the Court determined that gender-based discrimination should not limit women's rights to inheritance. (*C Masilamani Mudaliar & Ors v. Idol of Sri Swaminathaswamiswaminathaswami Thirukoil & Ors* (1996). http://judis.nic.in/supremecourt/qrydisp.asp?tfnm=16097)

In 2005, a local court in Zambia ruled that women married under customary law had the right to a share of marital property in the event of divorce or death of the husband. This decision was a landmark judgment, since women in customary marriages typically only receive marital property at the discretion of their ex-husbands or ex-husbands' families. ("ZAMBIA: Landmark judgment for women in customary marriages." IRINNews, December 21, 2005. http://www.irinnews.org/report.asp?ReportID=50812&SelectRegion=Southern_Africa)

References

COHRE, *Sources 5: Women and Housing Rights* (Centre on Housing Rights and Evictions 2000). http://www.cohre.org/lbframe.htm

Human Rights Watch, *Double Standards: Women's Property Rights Violations in Kenya* (Human Rights Watch 2003). http://www.africafocus.org/country/kenya_hrw.php

Kenya Commission on Human Rights, *From Despair to Hope: Women's Right to Own and Inherit Property* (Kenya Commission on Human Rights 2004). http://www.policyproject.com/pubs/countryreports/KEN_InheritanceRights.pdf

Mwenda, Kenneth K., Florence N. M. Mumba & Judith Mvula-Mwenda, *Property-Grabbing under African Customary Law: Repugnant to Natural Justice, Equity, and Good Conscience, Yet a Troubling Reality,* 37 Geo. Wash. Int'l L. Rev. 949–67 (2005).

OHCHR, *Convention on the Elimination of All Forms of Discrimination against Women,* Arts. 15, 16 (Office of the United Nations High Commissioner for Human Rights 1979). http://www.ohchr.org

Rwebangira, Magdalena K. & Maria B. Tungaraza, *Review and Assessment of Laws Affecting HIV/AIDS in Tanzania,* Chapter 7 (Tanzania Women Lawyers Association 2003). http://www.policyproject.com/pubs/countryreports/TZlawreview_sumbooklet.pdf http://www.policyproject.com/pubs/countryreports/TZlawreview.pdf (Full report)

Strickland, R. S., *To Have and to Hold: Women's Property and Inheritance Rights in the Context of HIV/AIDS in Sub-Saharan Africa* (International Center for Research on Women 2004). http://www.icrw.org/docs/2004_info_haveandhold.pdf

Tripp, A., *Women's Movements, Customary Law, and Land Rights in Africa: The Case of Uganda,* 7(4) African Studies Quarterly (2004). http://web.africa.ufl.edu/asq/v7/v7i4a1.htm

UNAIDS, UNFPA & UNIFEM, *Women and HIV/AIDS: Confronting the Crisis* (UNAIDS, United Nations Population Fund & United Nations Development Fund for Women 2004). http://womenandaids.unaids.org/publications.html

7.3 Marital Rape

The Issue

Marital rape is generally defined as unwanted intercourse obtained by a woman's husband or ex-husband through force, threat of force, or when she is unable to consent. Married women are at high risk for HIV in countries where transmission occurs primarily through heterosexual sex and cultural norms condone male promiscuity and/or patriarchal control of the married couple's sexual activity. Trauma and tissue tearing caused by forced sex can increase the likelihood of HIV transmission. Marital rape is currently underreported because of cultural norms, social stigma, and the fact that many countries lack a supportive justice system. While most countries do penalize rape, many create exceptions for forced marital sex. In India, for example, a husband who engages in nonconsensual sex with his wife is not guilty of rape if his wife is over the age of 15 (see also Topic 8.3).

Legal and Policy Considerations

A number of countries have criminalized marital rape in recent decades, adopting laws acknowledging that marriage does not signify an agreement to sexual intercourse at any time and that married women have the right to refuse sex with their husbands. In addition, members of the United Nations that have ratified the *Convention on Elimination of All Forms of Discrimination Against Women* (CEDAW) are obligated to enact laws prohibiting discrimination against women.

Criminalizing marital rape may help reduce HIV transmission by discouraging HIV-positive men from having forced sex with their uninfected wives. However, implementation of laws against marital rape requires certain considerations. For instance, consent for sex must be very clearly defined. Many current definitions of consent are too narrowly defined to account for the variety of situations in which women may find themselves.

Furthermore, laws against marital rape alone are not sufficient for protecting women from contracting HIV. Societal norms in many countries dictate that women are inferior to men, and customary law often does not recognize marital rape. Since women in such countries lack the power to negotiate sex and safer sex practices, laws that contribute to the marginalization of women must also be repealed or reformed in an effort to empower women against marital rape.

Practice Examples

In Mexico, the Supreme Court overturned a 1994 decision that characterized violently forcing a spouse to have sex as the exercise of a conjugal right. In a unanimous ruling, the court declared that forced sex within marriage is considered rape and is punishable by law. Elizabeth Malkin and Ginger Thompson. "Mexican Court Says Sex Attack by a Husband Is Still a Rape." *New York Times,* November 17, 2005.

In Zimbabwe, the *Sexual Offences Act* of 2001 considers nonconsensual sex within marriage as rape and criminalizes the willful transmission of HIV to another person. Section 16 of the Act provides a sentence of up to 20 years for an HIV positive person convicted of rape or sodomy, regardless of whether the individual is aware of his status. (*Sexual Offences Act (Act 8/2001)*. http://www.kubatana.net/html/archive/legisl/010817sexoff.asp?sector=LEGISL)

The Supreme Court of Nepal decided in 2002 that husbands who force their wives to have sex can be charged with rape. The court cited both international human rights obligations and religious texts in support of its decision. (*Forum for Women, Law and Development v. Ministry of Law,* 55 Nepali Sup. Ct. 2058 (2001–2002). http://www.fwld.org.np/marrape.html)

References

Dhaliwal, M., *Creation of an Enabling and Gender-Just Legal Environment as a Prevention Strategy for HIV/AIDS among Women in India,* 4(2/3) Canadian HIV/AIDS Policy & Law Newsletter (1999). http://www.aidslaw.ca/publications/publicationsdocEN.php?ref=230

Human Rights Watch, *Just Die Quietly: Domestic Violence and Women's Vulnerability to HIV in Uganda* (Human Rights Watch 2003). http://www.hrw.org/reports/2003/uganda0803/

Malkin, Elizabeth & Ginger Thompson, *Mexican Court Says Sex Attack by a Husband Is Still a Rape,* New York Times (November 17, 2005).

Mishra, S. & S. Singh, *Marital Rape: Myth, Reality, and Need for Criminalization,* Feminist Studies and Law Relating to Women, Criminal, Sexual Offences (Eastern Book Company 1998–2005). http://www.ebc-india.com/lawyer/articles/645.htm

OHCHR, *Convention on the Elimination of All Forms of Discrimination against Women* (Office of the United Nations High Commissioner for Human Rights 1979). http://www.ohchr.org

United Nations, *Declaration on the Elimination of Violence against Women* (United Nations 1993). http://www.unhchr.ch/huridocda/huridoca.nsf/(Symbol)/A.RES.48.104 .En?Opendocument

WHO, *World Report on Violence and Health* (World Health Organization 2002). http://www.who.int/violence_injury_prevention/violence/world_report/en/

7.4   Reproductive Rights

The Issue

Reproductive rights encompass individuals' freedom to determine the number, spacing, and timing of their children; the right to access the information necessary to make such determinations; and the right to the highest available standard of sexual and reproductive health. HIV-positive women face numerous barriers to the realization of these rights, including both laws and informal practices that restrict reproductive freedom. Many of these restrictions—such as forced or coerced sterilization, recommended abstinence from sex and childbearing, and compulsory HIV testing—are designed to prevent the birth of HIV-positive children. However, with access to appropriate reproductive health care, counseling and treatment, HIV-positive women are able to engage in sex and childbearing with minimal risk of transmission to their partners or infants.

Legal and Policy Considerations

Reproductive rights require governments to minimize restrictions on reproductive liberty and maximize access to resources that enhance autonomous reproductive decision-making. Many governments, with assistance from NGOs, have integrated HIV prevention into existing family planning and reproductive health services. Others have adopted the opposite approach, linking family planning counseling with existing HIV services. Few nations have reproductive policies that actively discriminate against women with HIV, though ostensibly neutral laws often produce discriminatory results. For example, in many African and Latin American countries, abortion is illegal. Although this applies to all women in those jurisdictions, it disproportionately affects HIV-positive women who (i) may be more likely to seek an abortion, or (ii) may experience greater physical risk if they opt to have an abortion illegally. Similarly, contraception access and education is inadequate in many countries, leaving HIV-positive women to choose between abstinence and the risk of transmitting the HIV virus.

Medical advances—particularly the ability to reduce dramatically mother-to-child transmission of HIV—have also raised new legal concerns in the area of reproductive rights (see Topic 1.2). Some countries with high HIV prevalence include routine ("opt-out") HIV testing as an element of prenatal care (see Topic 1.1). While this allows governments to pursue the valid public health goals of reducing transmission and connecting women to treatment, it may also reduce women's autonomy in an important area of reproductive health care. Without adequate education, counseling, and access to health care services (including affordable antiretroviral treatment and abortion services), knowledge of serostatus does little to advance HIV-positive women's reproductive choices.

Practice Examples

The Philippines Reproductive Health Program identified prevention and treatment of HIV and AIDS as a necessary element of the Reproductive Health Care Package available through government-funded health clinics. (Center for Reproductive Rights 2005)

South Africa's Constitution (adopted in 1996) specifically guarantees citizens' reproductive rights. Section 9(3) outlaws discrimination on the grounds of pregnancy; section 12(1)(c) states that everyone has the right "to be free from all forms of violence from both public and private sources." This clause guarantees bodily and psychological integrity, which specifically includes the right "to make decisions concerning reproduction" and "to security and control over bodies." Decisions concerning reproduction can include decisions related to family planning, pre-natal care, safe delivery and postnatal care, as well as prevention and treatment of reproductive tract infections, sexually transmitted diseases, and abortion. (http://www.polity.org.za/html/govdocs/constitution/saconst.html?rebookmark=1)

UNAIDS and UNFPA, together with other civil society groups and NGOs, issued the *New York Call to Commitment Linking HIV/AIDS and Sexual and Reproductive Health* in 2004. This statement reiterates the important linkages between HIV/AIDS and sexual and reproductive health, and the broader links between human rights and public health, calling on countries to improve education and access to services around sexual and reproductive health and the prevention and treatment of HIV. (http://www.unfpa.org/publications/detail .cfm?ID=195&filterListType=3)

References

Center for Reproductive Rights, *Pregnant Women Living with HIV/AIDS: Protecting Human Rights in Programs to Prevent Mother-to-Child Transmission of HIV* (Center for Reproductive Rights 2005). www.crlp.org/pdf/pub_bp_HIV.pdf

―――, *Women of the World: Laws and Policies Affecting Their Reproductive Lives in East and Southeast Asia* (Center for Reproductive Rights 2005).

―――, *Women of the World: Laws and Policies Affecting Their Reproductive Lives* (Center for Reproductive Rights, various). http://www.crlp.org

Cottingham, J., *Linkages between SRH and HIV/AIDS* (PowerPoint presentation at "Women and HIV/AIDS in CEE: Bringing Different Communities Together to Advance Common Goals," Warsaw, November 11–12, 2005). http://health.osf.lt/downloads/news/Cottingham.ppt

de Bruyn, M., *Reproductive Rights for Women Affected by HIV/AIDS?: A Project to Monitor Millennium Development Goals 5 and 6* (Ipas 2005). www.ipas.org/publications/en/MDGRR_E05_en.pdf

———, *HIV/AIDS and Reproductive Health, Sensitive and Neglected Issues: A Review of the Literature and Recommendations for Action* (Ipas 2005). www.ipas.org/publications/en/HIVLITREV_E05_en.pdf

OHCHR, *Convention on the Elimination of All Forms of Discrimination against Women,* Art. 12 (Office of the United Nations High Commissioner for Human Rights 1979). http://www.ohchr.org

UNAIDS, UNFPA, et al., *New York Call to Commitment Linking HIV/AIDS and Sexual and Reproductive Health* (United Nations Population Fund 2004). http://www.unfpa.org/publications/detail.cfm?ID=195&filterListType=3

UNFPA & WHO, *Sexual and Reproductive Health of Women Living with HIV/AIDS: Guidelines on Care, Treatment and Support for Women Living with HIV/AIDS and Their Children in Resource-Constrained Settings* (United Nations Population Fund & World Health Organization 2006). http://www.unfpa.org/publications/detail.cfm?ID=297

7.5 Sexual Harassment and Violence

The Issue

Gender violence and sexual harassment contribute to women's HIV risk through physiological, social, and economic pathways. HIV-transmission risk increases during violent or forced-sex situations, because abrasions caused by forced penetration facilitate entry of the virus. Research indicates that women who are beaten or dominated by their partners are much more likely to become infected by HIV due to their lack of power over their bodies and sexual lives. Fear of violence undermines women's ability to seek treatment. Finally, women who are victims of sexual harassment are more likely to engage in behaviors that place them at risk for acquiring HIV.

Legal and Policy Considerations

International human rights law obligates nations to ensure that women are not subjected to gender violence. The UN Committee on the Elimination of Discrimination against Women recommends that states implement legal measures, including penal sanctions, to protect women from all kinds of violence. Many states have responded by enacting legislation criminalizing rape, domestic abuse, and sexual harassment. However, because gender violence and sexual harassment encompass so many forms of abuse, no single legal or policy approach can protect women effectively and punish the perpetrators of the crimes. Indeed, the successful implementation of protection against sexual harassment and violence can be elusive in many societies where women are not socially or economically empowered to protect themselves.

Due to the trauma involved, gender violence crimes require sensitivity from personnel in the medical and legal professions. Some countries require training to sensitize law enforcement officials and members of the judiciary, while in others women must contend with institutionalized gender bias and discriminatory practices. These structural barriers often discourage women from reporting gender violence, and require affirmative state action to be overcome.

Practice Examples

South Africa has passed a number of progressive laws designed to prevent gender violence. The 1998 *Domestic Violence Act* criminalizes nonconsensual sex within marriage and violence in both marital and nonmarital relationships. The Act imposes duties on the police to provide necessary assistance, including arrangements for suitable shelter and medical treatment, to victims of domestic violence, as well as information about their rights; there are sanctions for noncompliance with these duties. South Africa also has established specialized sexual offenses courts that aim to reduce the trauma experienced by sexual assault complainants during the investigations and prosecution processes; to improve coordination among criminal justice agencies; and to increase the reporting, prosecution, and conviction rate for sexual offenses. (*Domestic Violence Act 116 of 1998.* http://www.info.gov.za/gazette/acts/1998/a116-98.pdf)

In the Philippines, the investigation of offenses committed against women must be handled by an all-female team of police officers, examining physicians, and prosecutors. Protective measures such as the right to privacy and closed-door investigations are accorded to the victim. (*Rape Victim Assistance and Protection Act of 1998-03-24*)

In Namibia, the *Combating of Domestic Violence Act* covers various forms of domestic violence, including sexual violence, harassment, intimidation, economic violence, and psychological violence. The law authorizes several alternatives to filing criminal charges against perpetrators of domestic violence. Those who have suffered violence may use a simple, free procedure to request a protection order from a magistrate's court, directing the abuser to stop the violence, prohibiting the abuser from having any contact with the victim, or ordering the abuser to leave the common home. Obtaining a protection order does not have to occur in lieu of bringing criminal charges against the abuser. Both actions can proceed simultaneously. In addition, the law contains provisions designed to protect the privacy of a complainant who brings a criminal charge and to make the court process less traumatic. (*Combating of Domestic Violence Act,* 2003. http://www.lac.org.na/grap/grapdomv.htm)

References

Amnesty International, *Women, HIV/AIDS, and Human Rights* (Amnesty International 2004). http://web.amnesty.org/library/Index/ENGACT770842004

Human Rights Watch, *Policy Paralysis: A Call for Action on HIV/AIDS-Related Human Rights Abuses against Women and Girls in Africa* (Human Rights Watch 2003). http://www.hrw.org/reports/2003/africa1203/9.htm#_Toc56508501

OHCHR, *Convention on the Elimination of All Forms of Discrimination against Women* (Office of the United Nations High Commissioner for Human Rights 1979). http://www.ohchr.org

Panos, *The Intimate Enemy: Gender Violence and Reproductive Health,* 27 Panos Briefing (1998). http://www.panos.org.uk/resources/reportdownload.asp?type=report&id=1028

UNDP, *Dying of Sadness: Gender, Sexual Violence and the HIV Epidemic* (United Nations Development Programme 1999). http://www.undp.org/hiv/publications/gender/violence.htm

UNICEF, *Domestic Violence against Women and Girls* (UNICEF 2000). http://www.unicef-icdc.org/publications/pdf/digest6e.pdf

WHO, *World Report on Violence and Health* (World Health Organization 2002). http://www.who.int/violence_injury_prevention/violence/world_report/en/

7.6   Traditional Practices

The Issue

In some traditional African communities the continued practice of wife inheritance and widow "cleansing" violates women's human rights and contributes to the spread of HIV. Wife inheritance occurs when the brother or nearest male relative of the deceased husband "inherits" the widow, and has the right to marry her, often against her will. Widow "cleansing" requires a widow to have unprotected sex with one of her husband's male relatives or a designated "cleanser," in order to exorcise her husband's spirit. While women theoretically can refuse to participate in these activities, in practice there is great social pressure to comply. Women who refuse risk theft of their land and property by in-laws, banishment from their communities, and other forms of social opprobrium.

Female circumcision (FC) is practiced primarily in certain countries in Africa and parts of the Middle East, where it carries great importance as a social ritual. Critics assail the practice on ethical and medical grounds, arguing that it violates women's dignity and bodily integrity and exposes them to serious health risks. Because FC is often performed in unhygienic conditions, with the same equipment used on many girls, it is thought that it may facilitate HIV transmission. Additionally, lasting damage to the genital area can increase the risk of HIV transmission during intercourse later in life. In many communities where FC is practiced, girls who refuse the procedure can suffer serious social consequences that significantly impair mental health and emotional well being.

Legal and Policy Considerations

A number of African countries operate under dual legal systems that recognize both customary and statutory law. Customary law consists of the indigenous customs of traditional communities, some of which—including wife inheritance and widow "cleansing"—promote the subordination of women. Nations that accord customary law the same weight as statutory law thus sanction such practices and eliminate women's opportunity to seek legal redress. Other countries elevate statutory law above customary law when the two bodies of law conflict, but confusion and bias among judicial officials can allow harmful traditional practices to continue. Discriminatory property laws (see Topic 7.2) also encourage wife inheritance by limiting widows' access to marital property, thereby increasing their economic dependence on male inheritors.

Some African countries have begun a process of legal reform in this area. For example, the Parliaments of Kenya and Zimbabwe considered bills in 2006 that would criminalize wife inheritance. However, a purely legal approach without adequate education and enforcement is unlikely to result in rapid abandonment of valued traditional practices. A complementary effort should be made to encourage tribal leaders to replace wife inheritance and widow "cleansing" with less risky rituals. There is some evidence demonstrating the effectiveness of such an approach.

FC may violate a number of recognized human rights protected by international instruments, including women's right to be free from discrimination, the right to physical integrity, the right to health, and the rights of the child. State parties to these instruments therefore have a duty to take steps to prevent or redress the practice of FC. Many countries have enacted statutes that specifically prohibit FC, whereas others have relied upon existing criminal codes that assign penalties to practices that can be interpreted to include FC. While such legislative action can have important practical and symbolic value, in many countries law enforcement mechanisms are weak and lack resources.

As an alternative to criminalization, some governments have adopted a medical approach that requires FC to be performed by trained personnel in sanitary clinical facilities. While this alleviates many of the health concerns associated with the practice, it does not address the ethical and human rights violations mentioned above. Furthermore, requiring medical personnel to perform FC may contravene professional codes of ethics.

Practice Examples

In Malawi, after unsuccessfully attempting to ban widow "cleansing," health officials convinced traditional leaders to encourage the use of condoms for those who are involved in the rituals. Some local tribal leaders have welcomed the initiative, modifying customary law to punish cleansers who force women to have sex without condoms (Ligomeka 2003).

In 2005, the government of Zambia amended the penal code to make it illegal for any person to engage in a harmful cultural practice such as widow "cleansing," or to encourage another person to engage in the practice. This national level law reform supports ongoing changes to policies and practices at the local levels. The AIDS Care and Prevention Department at Chikankata Hospital began promoting alternative ritualistic methods of sexual "cleansing" though a process of consultation with local chiefs. These consultations explored alternatives to ritualistic cleansing, such as nonsexual practices or protected (using condoms) sexual practices. Subsequently, the chiefs in the Chikankata Hospital area enacted a law to abolish ritual cleansing by sexual intercourse in the early 1990s.

In 1994, the Ministry of Health of Egypt issued a decree permitting only doctors in government hospitals to perform FC. Under pressure from women's rights and health advocates, the policy was reversed in 1995 and all licensed health professionals were banned from performing the procedure. In 1997 an Egyptian court overturned this ban, concluding that FC was a form of surgery that doctors have the legal "right" to perform. Supporters of the court ruling argued that prohibiting qualified medical personnel from practicing FC forced women to rely upon traditional practitioners and exposed girls to undue risk of injury and death. The matter was finally resolved in 1998, when Egypt's highest court rejected arguments that FC is a religious dictate authorized by the Koran and directed that authorities ban licensed health professionals from performing FC.

In the United States, several federal courts have granted asylum on the basis that the asylum seekers would be subjected to FC in their home countries: The Sixth Circuit Court of Appeals upheld fear of FC as a legitimate basis for a grant of asylum. *(Abay and Amare v. Ashcroft, 368 F.3d 634, 6th Cir. 2004).* The Ninth Circuit Court of Appeals determined that past FC constitutes "persecution" sufficient to support a claim for asylum. In addressing the requirement that asylum seekers must demonstrate a *continuing* risk of harm in their home country, the court compared FC to forced sterilization insofar as it disfigures a woman, causes long term health problems, and deprives her of a normal and fulfilling sexual life. *(Mohammed v. Gonzalez, 400 F.3d 785, 9th Cir. 2005)*

References

Brady, M., *Female Genital Mutilation: Complications and Risk of HIV Transmission,* 13(2) AIDS Patient Care and STDs 709–16 (1999).

Human Rights Watch, *Discrimination in Property and Inheritance Rights and HIV/AIDS,* in *Policy Paralysis: A Call for Action on HIV/AIDS-Related Human Rights Abuses against Women and Girls in Africa* (Human Rights Watch 2003). http://www.hrw.org/reports/2003/africa1203/5.htm

Ligomeka, B., *Traditional Practices transformed by AIDS* (Inter Press Service News Agency November 8, 2003). http://ipsnews.net/interna.asp?idnews=21001

Luke, N., *Widows and 'Professional Inheritors': Understanding AIDS Risk Perceptions in Kenya* (Paper presented at the Annual Meetings of the Population Association of America, Atlanta GA., May 2002). www.ssc.upenn.edu/Social_Networks/Level%203/Papers/PDF-files/luke-2002b.pdf

Malungo, J. R. S., *Sexual Cleansing (Kusalazya) and Levirate Marriage (Kunjilila mung'anda) in the Era of AIDS: Changes in Perceptions and Practices in Zambia,* 53(3) Social Science & Medicine 371–82 (2001).

Rahman, A. & N. Toubia (Editors), *Female Genital Mutilation: A Guide to Laws and Policies Worldwide* (Zed Books 2000).

Shell-Duncan, B., *The Medicalization of Female "Circumcision": Harm Reduction or Promotion of a Dangerous Practice?* 52(7) Social Science & Medicine 1013–28 (2001).

Toubia, N., *Female Genital Mutilation: An Overview* (World Health Organization 1998).

UNAIDS, UNFPA & UNIFEM, *Women and HIV/AIDS: Confronting the Crisis* (UNAIDS, United Nations Population Fund & United Nations Development Fund for Women 2004). http://womenandaids.unaids.org/publications.html

UNICEF, *Female Genital Mutilation and Cutting: A Statistical Exploration* (UNICEF 2005). http://www.unicef.org/publications/index_29994.html

————, *Changing a Harmful Social Convention: Female Genital Mutilation and Cutting* (UNICEF Innocenti Research Centre 2005). http://www.unicef-icdc.org/publications/

SECTION 8

Children

8.1   Orphans, Inheritance, Birth Registration, Caregivers

The Issue

In the countries most affected by AIDS, the orphan population has exploded, causing severe strains on the social fabric. UNAIDS and WHO have estimated that in 2006 some 2.1 million people died of AIDS in sub-Saharan Africa alone, nearly three-quarters of all AIDS deaths in that year. Since 1990 the number of children who lost one or both parents due to AIDS in that region increased from less than 1 million to about 12 million. Even if children do not lose one or both of their parents to the epidemic, if there is AIDS in the family, children are likely to suffer adverse consequences due to loss of family income and impoverishment. They may have to miss school in order to care for ill family members or to go to work to help support the family financially. They are also likely to receive reduced parental care and supervision, and to be exposed to stigma and discrimination. They may be infected with HIV themselves. Key legal issues directly relevant to children who have lost one or both parents relate to inheritance, birth registration, and alternative care.

Legal and Policy Considerations

UNAIDS discourages the term "AIDS orphans" as overly stigmatizing and implying that the child has AIDS, which may not be the case. It suggests the term "orphans or other children made vulnerable by AIDS" and includes in the term "orphan" children who have lost one parent. In a major recent paper, UNICEF uses the terms "children affected by AIDS" and "affected children" to refer to children living with HIV, children who have lost one or both parents to AIDS, and "vulnerable children whose survival, well-being or development is threatened or impacted by HIV and AIDS" (UNICEF 2006 at 13). From a legal perspective, use of the term "orphan" to refer to a child who has lost one parent may be confusing: national laws frequently define orphans as children who are parentless, and the state has different responsibilities for children without parents than for children with a surviving parent.

The *Convention on the Rights of the Child* does not deal directly with inheritance; however, its prohibition on discrimination with respect to property could be deemed to include property obtained by inheritance. In its General Comment on HIV/AIDS and the rights of the child, the Committee on the Rights of the Child vigorously supports the property and inheritance rights of children. Nondiscrimination with respect to property upon dissolution of marriage or death of the husband is also critically important to women (and their children), and protected under the

Convention on the Elimination of All Forms of Discrimination against Women. Still, in many traditional patriarchal societies, widows and children have no or limited inheritance rights, legally or de facto. A solid, enforceable legal framework on property rights and inheritance that safeguards the interests of widows and children not only protects these important rights but would be directly beneficial to the state as well: a World Bank study on Mozambique and Zimbabwe concluded that governmental legal support for effectuating inheritances properly would be more effective than cash transfers to destitute widows and children.

The right to inheritance can be bolstered by ensuring that children are registered at birth. Birth registration is often essential for a host of other legal protections as well or for ensuring access to public services. Despite the strong endorsement of the duty of governments to ensure an infant's registration immediately after birth in the *Convention on the Rights of the Child* (Art. 7.1), still too many children are not registered. UNICEF has reported that in the year 2000 less than one-third of all births were registered in sub-Saharan Africa.

A related issue is the status of children born out of wedlock and the need for appropriate legislation to ensure that those children's civil rights are not diminished. While this is not explicitly addressed in the *Convention on the Rights of the Child,* the inclusion of ". . . birth or other status" in its general anti-discrimination clause has been deemed to guarantee equal rights to children born out of wedlock. Some countries have taken a different view on the basis of Islamic law or other religious doctrines.

The extended family is the first line of defense when a child's parents die or when one parent dies and the surviving parent is unable to care for the offspring. The *Convention on the Rights of the Child* (Art. 5) and the legislation of many countries give legal backing to such arrangements. Failing such solution, the state is required to ensure alternative care, which the *Convention on the Rights of the Child* designates as foster care, *kafalah* under Islamic law, adoption, or placement in an institution (Art. 20). New arrangements born out of necessity, such as child-headed households under the general care of the community, are being created. All of these alternative care mechanisms are fraught with social complexities and legal issues. Governments should be encouraged to review their existing legislation and regulatory frameworks to ensure they are up-to-date and serving the best interests of the children.

Practice Examples

The Uganda Children Act bestows special rights and responsibilities on local governments to protect children's inheritances:

> "every local government council shall mediate in any situation where the
> rights of the child are infringed and especially with regard to the protection

of a child, the child's right to succeed to the property of his or her parents." (*The Uganda Children Act 1997,* as amended, 3. L. Uganda, Cap. 59 2000)

The Kenya Birth and Deaths Registration Act requires all births to be registered. In order to register as many births as possible, the registration service was decentralized down to the level of the smallest administrative units (sublocations) to ensure the registration of home births, and registration was made free of charge. (Committee on the Rights of the Child, Consideration of reports submitted by States parties under article 44 of the Convention. Initial reports of States parties due in 1992. Kenya, para. 151, Feb. 16, 2001)

The OECS (Organization of Eastern Caribbean States) Family Law Reform and Domestic Violence Project has prepared draft model legislation for the region on, inter alia, status of children, adoption, child protection, juvenile justice, and family court (OECS 2002 and Sealy-Burke 2006).

Malawi has adopted a National Plan of Action for Orphans and Other Vulnerable Children which includes, inter alia, the review and updating of legislation with respect to alternative care, monitoring of alternative care arrangements by the state, involvement of children in decision-making, and facilitating networks of parents trained in the rights and protection of children. (Government of Malawi, National Plan of Action for Orphans and Other Vulnerable Children 2005–2009, June 2005, cited in UNICEF 2006 at 28)

References

Alderman, Harold, *The Implications of Private Safety Nets for Public Policy: Case Studies of Mozambique and Zimbabwe* (World Bank 2001).

Committee on the Elimination of Discrimination against Women, *General Recommendation No. 21: Equality in Marriage and Family Relations* (13th Session 1994). http://www.un.org/womenwatch/daw/cedaw//recommendations/recomm.htm

OECS, *Report on Reform to Child Protection Laws in the OECS and Turks and Caicos Islands* (Secretariat, Organization of Eastern Caribbean States 2002). http://oecs.org

OHCHR, *Convention on the Elimination of All Forms of Discrimination against Women* (Office of the United Nations High Commissioner for Human Rights 1979). http://unohchr.ch

Sealy-Burke, Jacqueline, *Protecting Children Affected by AIDS in the Caribbean: Recommendations for Legal Reform* (World Bank 2006). http://www.worldbank.org/HIVAIDS

Subbarao, Kalanidhi & Diane Coury, *Reaching Out to Africa's Orphans: A Framework for Public Action* (World Bank 2004). http://www.worldbank.org/HIVAIDS

UNAIDS, *UNAIDS' Editors' Notes for Authors* (UNAIDS 2006). http://www.unaids.org

UNAIDS & WHO, *2006 Report on the Global AIDS Epidemic* (UNAIDS & World Health Organization 2006). http://www.unaids.org

————, *AIDS Epidemic Update,* Dec. (UNAIDS & World Health Organization 2006). http://www.unaids.org

UNICEF, *Implementation Handbook for the Convention on the Rights of the Child* (UNICEF 1998). http://unicef.org

————, *Africa's Orphaned Generations* (reprint, UNICEF 2004). http://unicef.org.

————, *The State of the World's Children 2005: Children under threat* (UNICEF 2004). http://unicef.org

————, *The State of the World's Children 2006: Excluded and Invisible* (UNICEF 2005). http://unicef.org

————, *Child Protection and Children Affected by AIDS* (UNICEF 2006). http://unicef.org

UNICEF & UNAIDS, *The Framework for the Protection, Care, and Support of Orphans and Vulnerable Children Living in a World with HIV and AIDS* (UNICEF 2004). http://unicef.org

van Bueren, Geraldine, *The International Law on the Rights of the Child* (Martinus Nijhoff Publishers 1995).

8.2 Discrimination in Education

The Issue

Education is indispensable for the full development of the person. In addition, education decreases the risk that children will be sexually exploited, experience unwanted pregnancy, or acquire sexually transmitted infections. Additional years of schooling have been shown to lower the risk of HIV infection in children. Schools may provide nutrition assistance to the most needy, and may be the only forum for a discussion of safe sex practices, contraception, and HIV/AIDS geared to the child's level of development and maturity.

However, stigma and uncertainty about HIV and AIDS often lead to discrimination in the education sector. Children may be refused access to school due to their perceived or actual HIV seropositive status, or that of their parent/s, or they may be required to leave after having been admitted. Within the education system they may face discrimination in the form of segregation, isolation, or differential and prejudicial treatment.

Legal and Policy Considerations

Education is a basic right, as recognized by the International Covenant on Economic, Social and Cultural Rights (Art. 13) and the Convention on the Rights of the Child (Art. 28). The general antidiscrimination clause proscribing discrimination on the basis of "other status" in both of these international agreements has been interpreted by the relevant treaty-monitoring bodies as forbidding discrimination on the basis of HIV status.

National constitutions in many countries guarantee a right to education and contain generally-applicable antidiscrimination provisions that can be relied upon to outlaw or to combat HIV-based discrimination in educational settings. In addition, there is a broad category of laws and policies that prohibit discrimination in the context of education generally. Despite the existence of these constitutional and statutory protections, states are often unable to effectively regulate de facto discrimination and stigma that occur in schools, or to properly monitor private educational institutions.

Some countries have adopted laws and policies that directly prohibit discrimination in education based on HIV status. Countries that adopt this approach typically define these protections within a national law or policy that covers multiple aspects of HIV and AIDS (see the Philippines and Cambodia examples below). These provisions may contain a range of specific protections: for example, students with actual, perceived, or suspected HIV infection may not be subjected to additional or more severe discipline, denied participation in school activities or lessons, isolated from other students, or deprived of generally available benefits or services. These HIV-specific laws may apply to educational institutions generally but sometimes may only apply to schools in the public sector or to schools that fall within formal, specified categories.

Practice Examples

In the Philippines, the *AIDS Prevention and Control Act of 1998* prohibits discrimination in schools. Under the Act, no educational institution "shall refuse admission or expel, discipline, segregate, deny participation, benefits or services to a student or prospective student on the basis of his/her actual, perceived or suspected HIV status." (http://www.doh.gov.ph/pnacwebsite/RA8504.pdf)

Article 37 of the Cambodia *Law on the Prevention and Control of HIV/AIDS* states: "No educational institution shall refuse admission or expel, discipline, isolate or exclude from gaining benefits or receiving services to a student on the basis of the actual, perceived or suspected HIV/AIDS status of that student or his/her family members." (http://www.ilo.org/public/english/protection/trav/aids/laws/cambodia1.pdf)

Macedonia's *HIV/AIDS National Strategy* states that children with HIV/AIDS must be fully integrated into normal educational and social activities. The Strategy mandates that these children have full access to public schools and that they are not subject to discrimination from their parents, teachers, and community members. (http://hivaidsclearinghouse.unesco.org/ev_en.php?ID=4523_201&ID2=DO_TOPIC)

The *National HIV/AIDS Policy* of Zimbabwe commands "freedom from discrimination in all spheres of life and the right to full access to health care, education and welfare support" for children with HIV. (Sec. 6.5. http://hivaidsclearinghouse.unesco.org/ev_en.php?ID=5289_201&ID2=DO_TOPIC)

References

AIDS Law Project & AIDS Legal Network, *HIV/AIDS and the Law: A Resource Manual,* Chapter 11 (3rd ed., AIDS Law Project & AIDS Legal Network 2003).

Bundy, D. & M. Gotur, *Education and HIV/AIDS: A Window of Hope* (World Bank 2002).

Human Rights Watch, *Future Forsaken: Abuses against Children Affected by HIV/AIDS in India* (Human Rights Watch 2004). http://hrw.org/reports/2004/india0704/FutureForsaken.pdf

———, *Letting Them Fail: Government Neglect and the Right to Education for Children Affected by AIDS* (Human Rights Watch 2005). http://hrw.org/reports/2005/africa1005/

Lawyers Collective, *Legislating an Epidemic: HIV/AIDS in India,* Chapter 4 (Universal Law Publishing Co. Pvt. Ltd. 2005).

OHCHR, *International Covenant on Economic, Social, and Cultural Rights,* Dec. 16 1966, 993 UNTS 3, Art. 13 (Office of the United Nations High Commissioner for Human Rights 1966). http://www.unhchr.ch/html/menu3/b/a_cescr.htm

————, *Convention on the Rights of the Child,* Nov. 20, 1989, 1577 U.N.T.S. 43, art. 28 (Office of the United Nations High Commissioner for Human Rights 1989). http://www.ohchr.org/english/law/pdf/crc.pdf

UNESCO, *Convention against Discrimination in Education* (United Nations Educational, Scientific, and Cultural Organization 1960). http://portal.unesco.org/education/en/ev.php-URL_ID=18443&URL_DO=DO_TOPIC&URL_SECTION=201.html

————, *The Impact of HIV/AIDS on Young People: Reviewing Research Conducted and Distilling Implications for the Education Sector in Asia,* Discussion Paper 1 (United Nations Educational, Scientific, and Cultural Organization 2002).

————, *Guidelines for inclusion: Ensuring Access to Education for All* (United Nations Educational, Scientific, and Cultural Organization 2005). http://unesdoc.unesco.org/images/0014/001402/140224e.pdf

————, *Final Communiqué* (Sixth Meeting of the High-Level Group on Education for All, Cairo, November 14–16, 2006). http://www.unesco.org/education/HLG2006/Communique22Nov.pdf

UNESCO & United Nations Committee on Economic, Social, and Cultural Rights, *Right to Education, Scope and Implementation* (United Nations Educational, Scientific, and Cultural Organization 2003). http://portal.unesco.org/education/en/file_download.php/71d965358b3bb1627077df3eb6335b4eScope+and+impl.pdf

UNICEF & UNAIDS, *HIV/AIDS and Education: A Strategic Approach* (UNICEF 2003). http://www.unicef.org/aids/files/Education_HIV.pdf

————, *The Framework for the Protection, Care and Support of Orphans and Vulnerable Children Living in the World with HIV and AIDS* (UNICEF 2004). http://www.unicef.org/aids

UNICEF & World Bank, *Education and HIV/AIDS: Ensuring Education Access for Orphaned and Vulnerable Children: Training Module* (UNICEF & World Bank 2002). http://www.schoolsandhealth.org/OVC/OVC_Training_Manual_English.pdf

United Nations, *Draft Convention on the Rights of Persons with Disabilities* (Ad Hoc Committee on a Comprehensive and Integral International Convention on the Protection and Promotion of the Rights and Dignity of Persons with Disabilities, Eighth Session, New York, August 14–25, 2006). http://www.un.org/esa/socdev/enable/rights/ahc8adart.htm

————, *Rights of Persons with Disabilities* (Ad Hoc Committee on a Comprehensive and Integral International Convention on the Protection and Promotion of the Rights and Dignity of Persons with Disabilities 2005). http://www.un.org/esa/socdev/enable/rights/

United Nations Committee on Economic, Social, and Cultural Rights, *General Comment No. 14, 2000: The Right to the Highest Attainable Standard of Health* (Office of the United Nations High Commissioner for Human Rights 2000). http://www.ohchr.org

United Nations Committee on the Rights of the Child, *General Comment No. 3, 2003: HIV/AIDS and the Rights of the Child* (Office of the United Nations High Commissioner for Human Rights 2003). http://www.ohchr.org

8.3   Sexual Abuse, Legal Age, Child Marriage

The Issue

Sexual abuse can lead directly to HIV infection of both girls and boys. Sexual abuse of children occurs in many different settings and to children of all social strata. Girls are especially susceptible to sexual abuse by older men. Some girls engage in sexual relations with older men for money or other forms of support and protection; these "sugar daddies," as they are frequently called, seek out younger girls because they believe that they are less likely to be HIV-positive. This belief in turn leads to a decrease in condom use and a greater risk of HIV infection and pregnancy for the girls. Related to the issue of legal age for consent to sexual relations is the question of child marriage, a matter of great cultural and religious sensitivity in some countries but one that may put young girls at greater risk of HIV infection.

Legal and Policy Considerations

Governments protect against child abuse through, inter alia, the enactment of statutory rape laws. Generally, these laws make it a crime to engage in sexual relations with a child below a stated age, even with the child's consent. Some countries, however, allow a defense of consent for sexual relations with children above a certain age (e.g., Grenada, if the child is 16 or older) while others only allow it in limited circumstances and/or for defendants below a certain age (e.g., Saint Lucia, if the defendant is under 21 and has not previously been charged with a similar offense). The *Convention on the Rights of the Child,* which has been adopted by all but two countries in the world, specifies that all persons under the age of 18 are children; the attendant lack of maturity and vulnerability justify the wide range of protections provided by the Convention. Nevertheless, statutory rape laws frequently put the age of consent below 18 and even go as low as age 12. Without specifying a universally applicable minimum age, the Committee on the Rights of the Child has stated that 13 is too low.

Statutory rape laws are frequently gender specific and may exclude boys or provide for different ages of consent for boys and girls. If different, the age of consent for girls is typically higher than for boys. Thus, young boys are frequently deprived of equal protection of the law.

Statutory rape laws may raise other questions. While it is imperative to protect vulnerable children from the advances of manipulative older partners (who are more likely to have had previous sexual partners), criminalizing consensual relationships between adolescents who are close in age may be problematic. Also, enforcement actions may serve as a pretext for violating the privacy of adolescents with regard to their sexual relationships.

Other legal and policy provisions that address sexual abuse are not as specific and do not hinge on legal age. These provisions reflect positions taken in international law and elsewhere that the elimination of child abuse is of critical importance. Many countries have enacted laws and policies that provide the government with authority to set up systems for reporting and monitoring of child abuse and linking these actions to HIV prevention initiatives.

A child marriage is any marriage in which one of the spouses is under the age of 18, but frequently the marriage is one of a girl child with an adult male. The practice of child marriages does not just raise legal and human rights issues with respect to the right to free and full consent to marry, as recognized by the Universal Declaration of Human Rights and related international law instruments. In the context of HIV, "[c]hild marriage removes the girls' ability to negotiate whether or not they want to *have* sex at all, much less negotiate *safe* sex . . ." (UNICEF 2006 at 20; emphasis in original).

Both the Committee on the Elimination of All Forms of Discrimination against Women (General Recommendation No. 21, para. 36) and the Committee on the Rights of the Child (General Comment No. 4, para. 20, applicable to both girls and boys) advocate the establishment of the age of 18 as the minimum age for marriage. Countries have addressed the issue of child marriage in different ways. Some countries have enacted legal provisions that set a minimum age for marriage. Some provide that children are legally considered adults when they marry, depriving them of legal protections that apply only to children. Many countries have enacted provisions that specifically ban child marriage, along with other traditional practices harmful to women and children. Finally, some nations have yet to ban the practice through law, and some that have banned the practice continue to allow it to occur.

Even in societies where child marriage and polygamy (frequently associated with the practice of child marriage) have been outlawed, these traditional practices often continue to occur. Some countries have attempted to increase enforcement of marriage age requirements by requiring birth or marriage registries to accurately record the age and marriage status of a potential child spouse. Education about HIV prevention targeted at girls who marry young is another approach adopted in some national policies.

Practice Examples

The *African Charter on the Rights and Welfare of the Child* requires ratifying countries to take specific legislative, administrative, social, and educational measures to protect children from sexual and other forms of abuse. The Charter recommends the establishment of monitoring units to provide support for children and the enactment of systems to ensure treatment and follow-up of victims of child abuse. (http://www1.umn.edu/humanrts/africa/afchild.htm)

The Malawi *National HIV/AIDS Policy* instructs the government to "strengthen and enforce existing legislation to protect children and young people against any type of abuse or exploitation." The Policy also urges the government to ensure that children have adequate information and education for preventing HIV; that counselors are trained to counsel abused children and provide them with sexual health information; and that youth centers are created to provide safe havens for children to successfully develop. (http://www.aidsmalawi.org.mw/contentdocuments/Malawi%20National%20HIVAIDS%20Policy.pdf)

In Kenya, Section 14 of the *Children Act* prohibits early marriage and other traditional practices likely to harm the child's development: "No person shall subject a child to female circumcision, early marriage or other cultural rites, customs or traditional practices that are likely to negatively affect the child's life, health, social welfare, dignity or physical or psychological development" (Government of Kenya 2002).

In India, a 2006 Supreme Court decision requires marrying couples to register their age and consent with local authorities, rules that are intended to create obstacles for child marriage. Furthermore, children married against their will can file a petition to nullify the marriage within two years of attaining majority status or by a guardian when the petitioner is a minor (Johnson 2006, p. 2).

References

African Union, *African Charter on the Rights and Welfare of the Child,* OAU Doc. CAB/LEG/24.9/49 (African Union 1990). http://www1.umn.edu/humanrts/africa/afchild.htm

AVERT, *Worldwide Ages of Consent* (AVERT accessed 04/13/2007). http://www.avert.org/aofconsent.htm

Government of Kenya, *Children Act,* Supplement 95, Act 8, Kenya Gazette (Jan. 4, 2002).

Human Rights Watch, *Suffering in Silence: The Links between Human Rights Abuses and HIV Transmission to Girls in Zambia* (Human Rights Watch 2002). http://www.hrw.org/reports/2003/zambia/

———, *Future Forsaken: Abuses against Children Affected by HIV/AIDS in India* (Human Rights Watch 2004). http://hrw.org/reports/2004/india0704/

International Center for Research on Women, *Child Marriage* (International Center for Research on Women 2003). http://www.icrw.org

Johnson, Jo, *Indian Court's Ruling Puts Bigger Obstacles in Path of Child Marriage,* Financial Times, Asia-Pacific 2 (Feb. 16, 2006).

Lawyers' Collective, *Legislating an Epidemic: HIV/AIDS in India,* Chapter 4 (Universal Law Publishing Co. Pvt. Ltd. 2003).

Rwebingira, Magdalena K. & Maria B. Tungaraza, *Review and Assessment of Laws Affecting HIV/AIDS in Tanzania,* Chapter 8 (Tanzania Women Lawyers Association 2003). http://www.policyproject.com/pubs/countryreports/TZlawreview_sumbooklet.pdf http://www.policyproject.com/pubs/countryreports/TZlawreview.pdf (Full report)

Sealy-Burke, Jacqueline, *Protecting Children Affected by AIDS in the Caribbean: Recommendations for Legal Reform* (World Bank 2006). http://www.worldbank.org/HIVAIDS

UNICEF, *Early Marriage: A Harmful Traditional Practice* (UNICEF 2005). http://www.unicef.org/publications/files/Early_Marriage_12.lo.pdf

————, *The State of the World's Children, 2006: Excluded and Invisible* (UNICEF 2005). http://www.unicef.org/sowc06/pdfs/sowc06_fullreport.pdf

————, *Child Protection and Children Affected by AIDS* (UNICEF 2006). http://bettercarenetwork.org

United Nations Committee on the Elimination of Discrimination against Women, *General Recommendation No. 21: Equality in Marriage and Family Relations* (13th Session, United Nations Committee on the Elimination of Discrimination against Women 1994). http:/www.unhchr.org

United Nations Committee on the Rights of the Child, *General Comment No. 3: HIV/AIDS and the Rights of the Child* (Office of the United Nations High Commissioner for Human Rights 2003). http://www.unhchr.org

————, *General Comment No. 4: Adolescent Health and Development in the Context of the Convention on the Rights of the Child* (Office of the United Nations High Commissioner for Human Rights 2003). http://www.unhchr.org

8.4 Sexual and Economic Exploitation

The Issue

Children orphaned or made vulnerable by HIV and AIDS are at heightened risk for all forms of sexual and economic exploitation. Forced to make money for their families or to survive on their own, children often engage in dangerous manual labor or commercial sex. UNICEF estimates that 1.2 million children are trafficked each year, most sold into prostitution or used as bonded labor. These exploited children are much more vulnerable to HIV infection due to the nature of their activities and their lack of power to protect themselves from infection. They also are unlikely to have the ability to access treatment once infected.

Legal and Policy Considerations

Several international agreements deal with the sexual exploitation of children. The UN *Convention on the Rights of the Child (CRC),* the UN *Optional Protocol to the Convention on the Rights of the Child on the sale of children, child prostitution, and child pornography,* the ILO *Convention on the Worst Forms of Child Labour,* and the *Protocol to Prevent, Suppress and Punish Trafficking in Persons, Especially Women and Children, Supplementing the United Nations Convention against Transnational Organized Crime* all prohibit the use of children in prostitution, unlawful sexual activity, and pornography. Consent of either the child or the family should be irrelevant in prosecuting these forms of sexual abuse.

Many countries have enacted legislation that criminalizes child trafficking, commercial sex, and other exploitative activities. Nevertheless, some countries do not sufficiently protect children from exploitation, and others prosecute children forced into commercial sex or other illegal activities even though they are victims of crime themselves.

A number of international conventions protect children against economic exploitation and dangerous child labor. The *Convention on the Rights of the Child* requires states to protect children from "performing any work that is likely to be hazardous or to interfere with the child's education, or to be harmful to the child's health or physical, mental, spiritual, moral, or social development" (Art. 32.1). The CRC obligates states to enact legislation regulating the minimum age for employment and hours and conditions of employment—a great many countries have implemented these protections. The ILO *Minimum Age Convention* sets the minimum age at 15 years in industrialized countries and 14 years in developing countries, though it provides for the possibility of exceptions for child labor in family settings and domestic service. Unfortunately, this exception for domestic service may place some children, especially girls, at heightened risk for trafficking, sexual exploitation, and sexual abuse, and therefore, HIV infection.

The types of child labor that many countries have committed themselves to eliminate under the *Worst Forms of Child Labour Convention* (ILO No. 182) are: "(a) all forms of slavery or practices similar to slavery, such as the sale and trafficking of children, debt bondage and serfdom and forced or compulsory labour, including forced or compulsory recruitment of children for use in armed conflict; (b) the use, procuring or offering of a child for prostitution, for the production of pornography or for pornographic performances; (c) the use, procuring or offering of a child for illicit activities, in particular for the production and trafficking of drugs as defined in the relevant international treaties; and (d) work which by its nature or circumstances in which it is carried out, is likely to harm health, safety or morals of children." (Art. 3)

Practice Examples

In Kenya, the *Children Act* safeguards against trafficking and sexual exploitation. Section 13 states that "A child shall be entitled to protection from physical and psychological abuse, neglect and any other form of exploitation including sale, trafficking or abduction by any person." Section 15 provides that "A child shall be protected from sexual exploitation and use in prostitution, inducement or coercion to engage in any sexual activity, and exposure to obscene materials" (Government of Kenya 2002).

Zimbabwe's *National HIV/AIDS Policy* states that, in order to protect children with HIV/AIDS from abuse, the government should promote "education and stronger enforcement of laws that prohibit the use of young girls for reparation or barter." (http://hivaidsclearinghouse.unesco.org/ev_en.php?ID=5289_201&ID2=DO_TOPIC)

The *National Policy on HIV/AIDS* of Nigeria provides that the Nigerian government's support of orphans and vulnerable children must include protection for children from "all forms of abuse including violence, exploitation, discrimination, trafficking, and loss of inheritance." (http://hivaidsclearinghouse.unesco.org/ev_en.php?ID=4239_201&ID2=DO_TOPIC)

References

Government of Kenya, *Children Act,* Supplement 95, Act 8, Kenya Gazette (January 4, 2002).

Human Rights Watch, *No Rest: Abuses against Child Domestics in El Salvador* (Human Rights Watch 2004). http.hrw.org

ILO, *Global Report 2006: The End of Child Labour, Within Reach* (International Labour Organization 2006). http://www.ilo.org/public/english/standards/ipec/about/globalreport/2006/index.htm

Children

Rau, B., *HIV/AIDS and Child Labour. A State-of-the-Art Review with Recommendations for Action, Synthesis Report,* 6 Working Paper (International Labour Organization 2000). http.ilo.org

UNICEF, *The State of the World's Children, 2006: Excluded and Invisible* (UNICEF 2005). http://www.unicef.org/sowc06/pdfs/sowc06_fullreport.pdf

———, *Child Protection Information Sheets,* May (UNICEF 2006). http://www.unicef.org/publications/index_34146.html

United Nations Committee on the Rights of the Child, *General Comment 3: HIV/AIDS and the Rights of the Child,* para. 36 (Office of the United Nations High Commissioner for Human Rights 2003). http://www.unhchr.ch/tbs/doc.nsf/(symbol)/CRC.GC.2003.3.En?OpenDocument

SECTION 9

Clinical Research

9.1 Nondiscrimination in Selection of Research Subjects

The Issue

To avoid discrimination, selection of subjects for participation in HIV/AIDS research must conform to legal and ethical principles of justice. These principles typically require that benefits and burdens of research be distributed in equitable ways. HIV/AIDS research findings may vary with factors such as race, genetics, gender, age, social status, or other sensitive individual characteristics. HIV tends to burden vulnerable populations disproportionately because of social, economic, or other factors.

Under principles of justice, researchers must strike a balance between (1) over-burdening vulnerable populations with the risks of research and (2) under representing such populations in the findings and benefits of research.

Research participants should not be selected on the basis of judgments of social worth, potential contribution to society, or lifestyle. Researchers must also be careful to avoid selecting subjects in a way that leads to under-representation of vulnerable populations (such as pregnant women or children) in research results.

Legal and Policy Considerations

Distinctions in the selection of research participants should be driven by substantive scientific research questions. For example, enrollment of participants should not be affected by their injecting drug use (IDU) unless the protocol addresses an HIV prevention issue that is specific to IDU. Research participants should not be selected because of easy availability or manipulability, nor should they be systematically excluded because of their vulnerable status. Research findings and other preventive or treatment benefits provided should potentially benefit the participant population.

All research protocols should be submitted to external ethical review boards for evaluation and approval (see Topic 9.5). To gain approval, a research protocol must (1) justify the selection criteria for subjects; (2) outline the anticipated benefits that will accrue to the participants and the population or community from which they are drawn; and (3) justify the exclusion of members of a group that may benefit from the research.

Practice Example

The UNAIDS *Ethical Considerations in HIV Preventive Vaccine Research* (2000) offers this advice:

- Guidance Point 4: "In order to conduct HIV vaccine research in an ethically acceptable manner, the research protocol should be scientifically appropriate, and the desired outcome of the proposed research should potentially benefit the population from which research participants are drawn. [T]he selection of the research population should be based on the fact that its characteristics are relevant to the scientific issues raised; and the results of the research will potentially benefit the selected population. In this sense, the research protocol should:
  - justify the selection of the research population from a scientific point of view
  - outline how the risks undertaken by the participants of that population are balanced by the potential benefits to that population
  - address particular needs of the proposed research population
  - demonstrate how the candidate vaccine being tested is expected to be beneficial to the population in which testing occurs, and
  - establish safeguards for the protection of research participants from potential harm arising from the research."

References

CIOMS, *International Ethical Guidelines for Biomedical Research Involving Human Subjects* (Council for International Organizations of Medical Sciences 2002). http://www.cioms.ch/frame_guidelines_nov_2002.htm

HPTN, *Ethics Guidance for Research* (HIV Prevention Trial Network 2003). http://www.hptn.org/Web%20Documents/EWG/HPTNEthicsGuidanceFINAL15April2003.pdf

UNAIDS, *Ethical Considerations in HIV Preventive Vaccine Research* (UNAIDS 2000). http://www.iavi.org/viewfile.cfm?fid=171

World Medical Association, *Declaration of Helsinki* (World Medical Association 2004). http://www.wma.net/e/policy/b3.htm

9.2 Informed Consent

The Issue

Informed consent, which stems from the ethical principle of respect for persons, is important to protect individuals from the harms of research. It is a process through which competent persons can choose freely whether to participate in research. Obtaining informed consent begins when a participant is first contacted about the study and only ends when the study is complete and participant risks have subsided. Informed consent involves ascertaining an individual's capacity to consent as well as adequately communicating relevant risks, benefits, and rights concerning the research.

In the context of HIV research, concerns about competency, language, literacy, or cultural barriers often arise. Obtaining informed consent may include consent to be tested for HIV and should be accompanied by pre- and posttest counseling. HIV vaccine research may require counseling about the need to take precautions to avoid contracting the infection. Physiological, psychological, and social risks associated with HIV-related research should be carefully explored and explained to participants in ways they understand. Potential benefits of participating in research should also be explained in a way that does not unduly influence an individual's choice.

Legal and Policy Considerations

Pursuant to the *Declaration of Helsinki* and corresponding legal norms, informed consent is generally required of any person who participates in research, which includes research involving data or biological samples from the participant. Informed consent must meet specific requirements to be valid. The person consenting must be competent. Certain information must be disclosed to the potential participant (e.g., the right to withdraw from the study, potential risks and benefits, or compensation for resulting harms). The consent must generally be documented in writing and renewed every time the research protocol is modified or extended. The entire informed consent process must be approved by an appropriate ethics board. For individuals who lack the capacity to consent (e.g., minors, mentally disabled), a legally-recognized representative may provide consent subject to additional safeguards.

Concerning international research, HIV research may have to adhere to the legal requirements for informed consent in the sponsoring and host countries. Special precautions must be taken to communicate effectively all the necessary information in a manner that is linguistically and culturally appropriate. In some cultures, informed consent from individuals may be supplemented by seeking the consent of a community or family leader. Community or familial consent does not supersede or replace an individual's own decision to participate.

Practice Example

Researchers in India examined women's understanding of informed consent issues related to HIV after receiving either standard counseling or counseling enhanced with visual aids in an antenatal clinic. The researchers found that women's understanding of informed consent issues (including the right to refuse, the meaning of a signature, the right to consult others, and the social risks of an HIV diagnosis) increased significantly from baseline levels when given enhanced counseling. The researchers used the following counseling enhancements to improve comprehension of informed consent issues (Sastry et al. 2004):

- Greater privacy for both group counseling and individual counseling.
- Posters illustrating the main topics placed in the Generalized Education and Counseling (GEC) rooms.
- Flipchart visuals, similar to the posters, used during individual counseling.
- All visuals developed included substantial input from the counselors.
- The visuals used bold colors and conveyed singular messages.
- The posters were created to provide informational cues to the counselor to promote and maintain regularity and standardization in presentation.
- The counselors completed further training in the use of the visuals.

References

CIOMS, *International Ethical Guidelines for Biomedical Research Involving Human Subjects* (Council for International Organizations of Medical Sciences 2002) http://www.cioms.ch/frame_guidelines_nov_2002.htm

Sastry, J, H. Pisal, S. Sutar, et al., *Optimizing the HIV/AIDS Informed Consent Process in India,* 2(28) BMC Med. (2004). http://www.biomedcentral.com/1741-7015/2/28

UNAIDS, *Ethical Considerations in HIV Preventive Vaccine Research* (UNICEF 2000). http://www.iavi.org/viewfile.cfm?fid=171

United States Department of Health and Human Services, *The Common Rule: U.S. Federal Policy for the Protection of Human Subjects,* 45 C.F.R. § 46 (Department of Health and Human Services 2005). http://www.hhs.gov/ohrp/humansubjects/guidance/45cfr46.htm

United States National Bioethics Advisory Commission, *Ethical and Policy Issues in International Research: Clinical Trials in Developing Countries,* vol. 1 (National Bioethics Advisory Commission 2001). http://www.georgetown.edu/research/nrcbl/nbac/clinical/Vol1.pdf

WHO, *Informed Consent Form Templates* (World Health Organization, accessed 04/1/2007). http://www.who.int/rpc/research_ethics/guidelines/en/index.html

9.3   Confidentiality

The Issue

Confidentiality of research subjects and their identifiable health data is an acute concern in HIV research. Grounded in legal, ethical, and human rights principles of autonomy (which includes privacy interests in the control of one's personal information), confidentiality is a safeguard against the harms from stigma and discrimination that can result from participating in HIV research, publicizing HIV serostatus, or identifying risk behaviors. Failing to protect confidentiality and privacy adequately deters individuals from participating in HIV research.

The acquisition and use of personal data relating to HIV is essential to advance the health of society through biomedical research, epidemiological studies, treatment, and prevention of HIV. However, there is a tension between the use of HIV data to promote the public's health and the individual's interests in privacy and nondiscrimination. Practitioners (e.g., health care providers, researchers, or public health officials) may justifiably access HIV data for laudable purposes, but they must also adhere to robust confidentiality and security measures.

Legal and Policy Considerations

Confidentiality of human subject research data is protected, in part, through the informed consent process (see Topic 9.2). Use or disclosure of identifying information may not occur generally unless a research subject (or his/her legal guardian) consents (or authorizes). Additional confidentiality protections approved by ethics boards assure that researchers limit use and disclosure of identifiable data to the minimum necessary to achieve the research goals. Ethics boards may also evaluate the adequacy of security measures (such as the use of technology) to protect subject privacy.

Additional balancing is needed for purely records-based HIV research. While ethics board review is necessary in all cases of research involving humans or their data, some legal schemes allow an ethics board to waive individual informed consent for records-based research if it concludes that there are only minimal risks to individuals that are outweighed by anticipated benefits.

In some cultures, community input or consent may be needed prior to the performance of HIV research. Underlying these requirements is the need to respect the privacy (and other) interests of the community as distinct from the confidentiality rights of individuals.

Practice Example

Council of Europe, *Recommendation No. R (97) 5 of the Committee of Ministers to Member States on the Protection of Medical Data,* 1997, part 12 "Scientific Research," states:

"12.1. Whenever possible, medical data used for scientific research purposes should be anonymous. . . .

12.2. However, if such anonymisation would make a scientific research project impossible, and the project is to be carried out for legitimate purposes, it could be carried out with personal data on condition that:

a. the data subject has given his/her informed consent for one or more research purposes; or

b. when the data subject is a legally incapacitated person incapable of free decision, and domestic law does not permit the data subject to act on his/her own behalf, his/her legal representative or [another legal] authority . . . has given his/her consent in the framework of a research project related to the medical condition or illness of the data subject; or

c. disclosure of data for the purpose of a defined scientific research project concerning an important public interest has been authorised by the body or bodies designated by domestic law, but only if: (i) the data subject has not expressly opposed disclosure; (ii) despite reasonable efforts, it would be impracticable to contact the data subject to seek his consent; and (iii) the interests of the research project justify the authorisation; or

d. the scientific research is provided for by law and constitutes a necessary measure for public health reasons."

References

Council of Europe, *Recommendation No. R (97) 5 of the Committee of Ministers to Member States on the Protection of Medical Data* (Council of Europe 1997). http://www1.umn.edu/humanrts/instree/coerecr97-5.html

European Union, *Directive on the Protection of Individuals with Regard to the Processing of Personal Data and on the Free Movement of Such Data,* Council Directive 95/46, 1995 O.J. (L 281) 31 (European Union 1995). http://europa.eu.int/eur-lex/pri/en/oj/dat/2002/l_201/l_20120020731en00370047.pdf

United States Department of Health and Human Services, *U.S. Privacy Rule (HIPAA Privacy Rule), 45 C.F.R. §§ 160, 164* (United States Department of Health and Human Services 2003). http://www.hhs.gov/ocr/hipaa/finalreg.html

9.4 Equitable Access to Information and Benefits

The Issue

Principles of justice and international human rights require equitable access to information and benefits of HIV research. Participants in research, whether in the experimental or control arm, must have equal access to treatments demonstrated by the research as beneficial. A more difficult issue is the extent to which such treatments must be made more widely available in the host country. Failing to make such benefits available to the population that bore the risks of research is considered exploitive and inequitable. Whether the responsibility to provide interventions falls on the research sponsor or host country's national government, or both, is less clear.

Another issue stemming from the principle of justice is whether participants in international research should be treated similarly regardless of where the research is conducted or whether it is sufficient that participants be treated similarly to others in their country. Ideally, participants would be given access to the best care available anywhere in the world whether they are in developing or developed countries. Though recognized in leading international ethical guidelines, this high standard of care is not required. Instead, some recommend a middle standard: the highest level of care available in the host country. Others recognize a lower standard: the level of care currently provided by the public health system in the host country. Debate continues about what standard of care is ethically required.

Legal and Policy Considerations

Because many of the concerns about equitable access to benefits and information involve international HIV research, policy recommendations often emphasize capacity building in the host country. The host country must have a system to conduct independent ethical review of research. Proposed research should be separately reviewed and approved by both the sponsor's and host country's ethics boards, consistent with the following considerations:

- Researchers must evaluate a host country's capacity to provide interventions shown to be beneficial by the research, evaluate the possibility of providing interventions to a broader population, and provide justification for conducting research in a host country that cannot provide proven therapeutic benefits to a wider population;
- Researchers must propose how the research will improve the local expertise, facilities, and delivery capacity as well as what steps will be taken to assure sustainability;

175

- Researchers must define the time frame that therapeutic intervention will be provided to research participants once research is completed; and
- Researchers must define the standard of care that will be provided to research participants.

Practice Example

Nuffield Council on Bioethics' Report: *The Ethics of Research Related to Healthcare in Developing Countries.*

"9.48 [T]he following issues [should be] clearly considered by researchers, sponsors, national healthcare authorities, international agencies and research ethics committees as part of any research protocol before research relating to healthcare involving the testing of new interventions is undertaken:

- the need where appropriate to monitor possible long-term deleterious outcomes arising from the research, for an agreed period of time beyond the completion of the research;
- the possibility of providing participants with the intervention shown to be best (if they are still able to benefit from it), for an agreed period of time;
- the possibility of introducing and maintaining the availability to the wider community of treatment shown to be successful.

9.49 . . . [R]esearch proposals submitted to those committees should include an explanation of how new proven interventions could be made available to some or all of the host country population and that investigators should justify to the relevant research ethics committee why the research should be carried out if this is not thought possible."

References

CIOMS, *International Ethical Guidelines for Biomedical Research Involving Human Subjects* (Council for International Organizations of Medical Sciences 2002). http://www.cioms.ch/frame_guidelines_nov_2002.htm

Nuffield Council on Bioethics, *The Ethics of Research Related to Healthcare in Developing Countries* (Nuffield Council on Bioethics 2002). http://www.nuffieldbioethics.org/go/textonly/ourwork/developingcountries/publication_309.html

UNAIDS, *Human Rights and Ethical Perspectives on HIV/AIDS Vaccine Trials,* Issue Paper (Global Reference Group on HIV/AIDS and Human Rights, UNAIDS 2003). http://data.unaids.org/Topics/Human-Rights/hr_refgroup2_04_en.pdf?preview=true

9.5   Ethics Boards

The Issue

Ethics boards (also called Institutional Review Boards, or IRBs) review all proposed research protocols and ongoing research involving human participants or their identifiable data to safeguard the welfare and rights of participants and their communities. Ethics boards operate independently of research sponsors and economic, political, or professional influences to avoid conflicts of interest or bias in ethical evaluation. Board members should reflect competence in the field, multidisciplinary viewpoints, local and cultural fluency, diversity in age and gender, and lay perspectives.

The dual objectives of assuring ethical practice of research and minimizing harms to research participants and communities must be balanced with the need to further important research goals without undue hindrance or delay. Scientific review is an essential precondition of ethical research. Participants should not be exposed to risk unless the research has potential for demonstrable scientific benefit to humans. In some cases, ethics boards may also adjudge the scientific soundness of research studies, although such review may also be reserved to distinct scientific review boards. In international research, ethics board review and approval must occur in the country where the research is conducted, but may also be required by the sponsor country or organization.

Legal and Policy Considerations

Legal and policy guidelines for ethical review of HIV research studies in many countries set requirements concerning (1) membership on ethics boards, (2) terms of appointment and organization of the board, (3) operating procedures, (4) instructions for research applicants for ethical review, (5) decision-making authority of the board, and (6) substantive elements of ethical review subject to board approval.

Substantive elements that an ethics board must review typically include: study design, participant selection, anticipated risks and benefits, standards of care and protection of participants, informed consent or authorization processes, confidentiality and privacy measures, and community considerations. Many ethics boards have special processes for expedited review, waiver of any of the substantive elements (such as informed consent in records-based research), or research on vulnerable populations (e.g., children, mentally disabled people).

Practice Example

Indian Council of Medical Research, *Ethical Guidelines for Biomedical Research on Human Subjects*. Section on Ethical Review Procedures:

"The basic responsibility of an [Institutional Ethics Committee] is to ensure a competent review of all ethical aspects of the project proposals received and execute the same free from any bias and influence that could affect their objectivity. IECs should provide advice to the researchers on all aspects of the welfare and safety of the research participants after ensuring the scientific soundness of the proposed research through appropriate Scientific Review Committees. In smaller institutions the Ethics Committee may take up the dual responsibility of Scientific and Ethical Review. It is advisable to have separate Committees for each, taking care that the scientific review precedes the ethical scrutiny. The scientific evaluation should ensure technical excellence of the proposed study.

The IECs should specify in writing the authority under which the Committee is established, membership requirements, the terms of reference, the conditions of appointment, the offices and the quorum requirements. The responsibilities of an IEC can be defined as follows: (1) To protect the dignity, rights and well being of the potential research participants; (2) To ensure that universal ethical values and international scientific standards are expressed in terms of local community values and customs; and (3) To assist in the development and the education of a research community responsive to local health care requirements."

References

Nuffield Council on Bioethics, *Issues to Be Considered When Reviewing Research Proposals,* Appendix 3 in *The Ethics of Research Related to Healthcare in Developing Countries* (Nuffield Council on Bioethics 2002). http://www.nuffieldbioethics.org/go/textonly/ourwork/developingcountries/publication_309.html

Indian Council of Medical Research, *Ethical Guidelines for Biomedical Research on Human Subjects* (Indian Council of Medical Research 2000). http://www.icmr.nic.in/ethical.pdf

South African Medical Research Council, *General Principles,* Book 1 in *Guidelines for Ethics in Medical Research,* 4th edition (South African Medical Research Council 2002). http://www.sahealthinfo.org/ethics/book1.htm

WHO, *Operational Guidelines for Ethics Committees that Review Biomedical Research* (World Health Organization 2000). http://www.who.int/tdr/publications/publications/ethics.htm

SECTION 10

Information

10.1 Informational and Educational Material; Censorship

The Issue

The public availability and accessibility of scientifically accurate informational and educational materials is vital to efforts to prevent HIV transmission, link infected persons with health care and other services, and reduce the stigma and discrimination often directed at PLHIV and their families. Informational and educational materials should be widely accessible to all persons to ensure effective dissemination, available in languages understood by communities, and respectful of cultural traditions. Information should not perpetuate stereotypes, enable discrimination, or avoid explicit discussion of sensitive topics such as sex and drug use.

Censoring information related to HIV/AIDS is a common occurrence that can have detrimental effects on outreach programs, thwart the implementation of effective HIV prevention strategies, and exacerbate social stigma against HIV-positive persons. Critics of providing greater access to education and information programs insist that unrestricted information on certain prevention and awareness practices equals government support for dangerous or disfavored lifestyles. These critics may oppose, for example, information about condoms and sterile injection equipment on the theory that this information encourages behaviors such as promiscuous sex and injecting drug use. However, evidence demonstrates that these fears are unfounded, and that increased knowledge about a range of HIV-related issues is important to make HIV prevention and treatment programs a success and to protect against discrimination.

Legal and Policy Considerations

National laws and policies often require information to be disseminated as a component of HIV prevention and treatment programs. Some countries have created laws or policies that mandate the dissemination of specific information (e.g., how HIV is transmitted; effective prevention techniques; access to testing, counseling, and treatment) while others more generally endorse the importance of this information and encourage educational materials to be made widely available.

Countries have enacted laws and policies that guarantee access to this information and often disseminate it in cooperation with NGOs, multinational organizations, and local secular and religious leaders. These cooperative efforts may be difficult to achieve in some countries or regions due to resistance from groups who still harbor a distrust of outsiders, based upon past mistreatment and cultural insensitivity. In addition, these groups may be reluctant to support informational or educational campaigns that conflict with their religious, moral, or practical worldview. Also, international aid may be conditioned on the advancement or avoidance of certain messages, giving donors significant control over the content of prevention messages that reach the population.

In many countries, censorship of HIV and AIDS information is used as a tool for political gain or to enforce moralistic viewpoints on the appropriateness of common behaviors. Governments that censor information about the use of condoms and other safer sex practices, the benefits of using sterile injecting equipment, or the risks of contracting or transmitting HIV infection through various activities may undermine the effectiveness of HIV prevention efforts. In some cases, laws against obscenity prevent public health officials and NGOs from talking about sexual issues. While proponents argue these provisions should apply to HIV information to protect children and others against explicit sexual content, the release of accurate information is the best way to counter stereotypes and eliminate dangerous practices. Some countries have provided for exceptions to censorship laws for educational or scientific material that covers HIV information.

Practice Examples

Brazil has achieved significant success in containing the country's HIV epidemic by combining treatment and access strategies with comprehensive HIV prevention campaigns. These campaigns use explicit messages, multiple forms of media, and in many cases are targeted to specific at-risk groups (Okie 2006).

The complicated relationship between law and practice is illustrated by the Philippines *AIDS Prevention and Control Act 1998* and its implementation. The Act devotes several sections to education and information, requiring government personnel, teachers, health services workers, employers and others to provide information on HIV prevention, modes of transmission, treatment, and related issues. The Act differentiates the types of information to be provided and the approaches used based upon the setting: health care and workplace settings must include information about confidentiality; community education campaigns should incorporate the input of NGOs and community organizations. The Act requires information about HIV to be provided with all prophylactics and imposes penalties on those distributing misleading information related to HIV or AIDS. One limitation of the Act is that it requires that materials used in the education setting not to utilize sexually explicit materials or propagate birth control. (http://www.doh.gov.ph/pnacwebsite/RA8504.pdf) In practice, evidence demonstrates that access to information about condoms is further limited by contrary local laws, misinformation, and human rights abuses. (http://hrw.org/reports/2004/philippines0504/)

References

Human Rights Watch, *Unprotected: Sex, Condoms and the Human Right to Health* (Human Rights Watch 2004). http://hrw.org/reports/2004/philippines0504/

Okie, S., *Fighting HIV: Lessons From Brazil*, 354 New Eng. J. Med. 1977–81 (2006). http://content.nejm.org/cgi/content/full/354/19/1977

UNAIDS & IPU, *Handbook for Legislators on HIV/AIDS, Law and Human Rights: Action to Combat HIV/AIDS in View of its Devastating Human, Economic, and Social Impacts* (UNAIDS & Inter-Parliamentary Union 1999). www.ipu.org/PDF/publications/aids_en .pdf

UNAIDS & OHCHR, *International Guidelines on HIV/AIDS and Human Rights*, 2006 Consolidated version (UNAIDS & Office of the United Nations High Commissioner for Human Rights 2006). http://data.unaids.org/Publications/IRC-pub07/JC1252-InternGuidelines_en.pdf?preview=true

10.2   Regulation of NGOs

The Issue

Nongovernmental organizations (NGOs) are vital to providing services and information to their constituencies affected by HIV and AIDS. NGOs have proliferated around the world and serve multiple roles, including providing a voice for vulnerable and marginalized populations; advocating for law and policy changes; working with national and local governments, international organizations, funders, and independently to provide services to the population; and holding governments accountable for failing to address the HIV epidemic adequately. Many NGOs have developed close links with poor and underserved communities most adversely affected by HIV, and demonstrated an ability to reach out to people, to work in inaccessible areas, and to innovate, or in other ways achieve results that are difficult for official agencies.

While governments often have supportive, collaborative relationships with NGOs, in some instances NGOs and governments do not coexist well, particularly when NGOs criticize the government or represent disfavored groups. NGOs that support the rights of sex workers, homosexuals, and drug users may antagonize the government by advocating for policies that violate the law. Many governments have implemented widespread regulation of NGOs. Regulations may restrict the activities, expressions, and positions of NGOs, with implications for how they address the impact of HIV in their targeted constituencies.

Legal and Policy Considerations

In regulating NGOs, governments generally have tried to balance regulation and facilitation so that scarce government resources need not be committed to managing a complex regulatory framework for HIV/AIDS programs. While some countries have attempted to impose harsh restrictions on NGOs, others have developed a system of self-governance. NGOs may face three regulatory hurdles imposed under law: a restrictive system of registration; a requirement that government agencies administer and police their daily work; and requirements regulating agency funding, often mandating that funds be routed through or monitored by government agencies. These regulations may restrict the presence and activities of organizations that may be a source of aid and information to local communities that receive little or no help from their government. Governments without an open democratic tradition are more inclined to control and restrict NGOs, or even deny their right to exist. State agencies have been known to shut down HIV/AIDS NGOs for being too outspoken or critical of government policies.

Furthermore, some governments have gone as far as prosecuting educators working with NGOs for aiding and abetting illegal activities when they provide information about safer sex or drug injecting.

Governments may have legitimate reasons to regulate NGOs. The proliferation of NGOs, particularly around issues of HIV/AIDS, has resulted in a sometimes-confusing patchwork of programs. Even well-meaning NGOs may provide misleading or ideologically biased information; lack resources, technical skills, or experience; or attempt to impose strategies on local populations without accounting for their cultural traditions or best interests. NGO programs also may compete with similar government programs or monopolize funding for HIV outreach and prevention efforts.

More troubling is when government officials use regulation of NGOs and other community groups as a pretext for discrimination against certain segments of the population or to restrict the availability of informational and educational resources. Marginalized groups may depend on NGOs as their only effective advocates and their only source of credible information about HIV and AIDS. Onerous regulation that restricts the expression and association activities of NGOs and other community groups violates human rights and may have significant detrimental effects on HIV prevention and treatment efforts.

Practice Examples

The government of Mozambique has mandatory registration for foreign but not local NGOs. A law, *Decree 55/98,* regulates the registration and activities of foreign NGOs. The preamble to the law justifies the need for the establishment of a legal framework for foreign NGOs because of their complementary role to government initiatives in rehabilitation and development. According to the law, foreign NGOs must work for the creation of capacity within the Mozambican partner organizations and thereby ensure the sustainability of their activities. The partner organization and the foreign NGO must verify that no Mozambican has the necessary qualifications before an expatriate may be hired. While there is no mandatory registration for local NGOs, a large percentage do register with the Ministry of Justice, apparently because registration ensures greater donor funding.

The Philippines *AIDS Prevention and Control Act 1998* implements a robust education and information strategy, requiring information on HIV prevention, modes of transmission, treatment, and related issues to be provided in the community. The Act requires that community education campaigns should incorporate the input of NGOs and community organizations. However, it is unclear whether this cooperative approach has occurred in practice. (http://www.doh.gov.ph/pnacwebsite/RA8504.pdf)

In Brazil, HIV prevention programs have made aggressive efforts to reach sex workers (including by organizing national sex worker conferences) and men who have sex with men with HIV information and instructions on how to use condoms and negotiate condom use with partners. Broader messages to the general population were conveyed through the mass media and with the cooperation of NGOs to "humanize" the disease and fight stigma and discrimination. Individuals and groups from the most affected communities also played a major role, supported by local or national governments. The programs have been successful in reducing HIV transmission (Okie 2006).

The NGO Durbar Mahila Samanwaya Committee took over the management of the successful and well-known Sonagachi Project (an integrated STD/HIV intervention program for sex workers in Kolkata, formerly Calcutta) from a government public health institute in 1992. Since then, it has expanded its base (now representing some 65,000 sex workers in West Bengal) and its activities, including advocacy for workers' rights and operation of a microcredit scheme run by and for sex workers. (http://www.durbar.org)

References

Clark, J., *The Relationship between the State and the Voluntary Sector* (Global Development Research Center 1993). http://www.globalpolicy.org/ngos/state/relationship.htm

Honey, Mary, *Guide to the Nonprofit Organisations (NPO) Act* (NPO Legal Support Project, Legal Resources Center 1997). http://www.etu.org.za/toolbox/docs/building/guide.html

Lawyers' Collective, *Legislating an Epidemic: HIV/AIDS in India* (Universal Law Publishing Co. Pvt. Ltd. 2003).

Okie, S., *Fighting HIV: Lessons From Brazil*, 354 New Eng. J. Med. 1977–81 (2006). http://content.nejm.org/cgi/content/full/354/19/1977

SECTION 11

Access to Medicines

11.1   Patented and Generic Drugs: Overview

The Issue

Many World Bank-supported projects finance antiretroviral medicines (ARVs) and other drugs for HIV-related treatment. ARVs are expensive drugs, although competition from generics has helped to drive prices down. In countries where ARVs (and other relevant drugs) are patented, can generic drugs be manufactured or imported legally?

Legal and Policy Considerations

A patent is an exclusive right granted for an invention. It provides the patent owner with the legal means to prevent others from making, using, selling or importing the new invention for a limited period of time (usually 20 years). Patents are intended to provide incentives for innovative activity and are granted under national law. There are no "worldwide patents." For the 150 member countries of the World Trade Organization (WTO), the Agreement on Trade-Related Aspects of Intellectual Property Rights (TRIPS), and WTO decisions with respect to that agreement provides a common set of requirements.

The World Health Organization (WHO) favors the term "multisource pharmaceutical product" over the term "generic product" because the latter can have different meanings depending on context and jurisdiction. Under the WHO's definition, a generic drug is a "pharmaceutical product, usually intended to be interchangeable with the innovator product, which is usually manufactured without a license from the innovator company and marketed after expiry of the patent or other exclusivity rights." Further, "[g]eneric products may be marketed either under the approved nonproprietary name or under a brand (proprietary) name. They may be marketed in dosage forms and/or strengths different from those of the innovator products." (See References, Marketing Authorization of Pharmaceutical Products with Special Reference to Multisource (Generic) Products at 35.)

Whether a generic ARV can be manufactured or imported legally depends on the patent situation in the country. If there is a patent law that allows for the patenting of pharmaceutical products and if a given ARV is under patent, a generic version may only be manufactured or imported legally if: (a) there is an exception that can be invoked under national law, or (b) if the patent holder has voluntarily entered into a licensing agreement or has agreed not to enforce a patent.

A compulsory license is an authorization by the government to a third party or to itself (referred to as government use) to produce the patented product or to utilize the patented process without the consent of the patent owner (with appropriate remuneration to the patent owner). National laws should provide the option of compulsory licensing for (but not limited to) cases of national emergency or circumstances of extreme urgency. The HIV epidemic can qualify as such a situation. Other grounds for compulsory licenses may be to remedy anticompetitive practices, for public noncommercial use (specifically mentioned in Art. 31 TRIPS Agreement), or to enable the use of a dependent patent. There are special considerations for compulsory licensing for WTO Members (see Topic 11.2).

A generic pharmaceutical producer may seek a compulsory license from the government to manufacture or import ARVs or the procurement authority may invoke legislation that permits government use of third party patents. Many national patent systems also include an exception for testing of generic drugs for purposes of marketing approval before patent protection expires. This exception is sometimes called a "regulatory review" or "Bolar" exception. Other typical exceptions include exceptions for research or for experimental use.

Practice Example

In 2003, the Malaysian government authorized a local company to import three ARVs. The Minister of Domestic Trade and Consumer Affairs authorized the company to import generic versions of the medicines from India, for the sole purpose of supplying public hospitals. In the authorization letter, the Minister relied on Section 84 of the *Malaysian Patents Act*. The cited provision allows the Minister to authorize a government agency or third person to exploit a patented invention in the case of a national emergency or where the public interest so requires. The authorization contained specific terms and conditions with regard to price, differentiation in shape and color from the patented product, and labeling of the medicines. The Ministry of Health reported a significant reduction in monthly costs of treatment as a consequence of the introduction of the generic ARVs.

References

Musungu, Sisule F. & Cecilia Oh, *The Use of Flexibilities in TRIPS by Developing Countries: Can They Promote Access to Medicines,* Case Study 4C, August (Commission on Intellectual Property Rights, Innovation, and Public Health, World Health Organization 2005). http://www.who.int/intellectualproperty/studies/TRIPS_flexibilities/en/index.html

Tayler, Yolanda, ed., *Battling HIV/AIDS: A Decision Maker's Guide to the Procurement of Medicines and Related Supplies,* Chapter 2 in *Intellectual Property Rights: A Concise Guide* (World Bank 2004). www.worldbank.org/aids

———, ed., *Intellectual Property Rights,* Annex B in *Intellectual Property Rights: A Concise Guide* (World Bank 2004). www.worldbank.org/aids

WHO, *Marketing Authorization of Pharmaceutical Products with Special Reference to Multi-source (Generic) Products: A Manual for a Drug Regulatory Authority,* 5 Regulatory Support Series, WHO/DMP/RGS/98.5 (World Health Organization 1999).

WIPO, *FAQs on Patents* (World Intellectual Property Organization, accessed 04/13/2007). http://www.wipo.int/patentscope/en/patents_faq.html#patent

World Bank, *Intellectual Property: Balancing Incentives with Competitive Access,* Chapter 5 in *Global Economic Prospects 2002: Making Trade Work for the World's Poor* (World Bank 2002).

11.2   WTO Members: Special Considerations under the TRIPS Agreement

The Issue

Although patent law is a matter of national legislation, WTO member countries need to adapt national law to TRIPS requirements to avoid being challenged under WTO dispute settlement rules.

Legal and Policy Considerations

Member countries of the World Trade Organization (WTO) are bound by the requirements of the *Agreement on Trade-Related Aspects of Intellectual Property Rights* (TRIPS Agreement or TRIPS). The TRIPS Agreement contains comprehensive minimum standards in various areas of intellectual property, including patent protection.

The TRIPS Agreement requires WTO members to establish, among other things, basic criteria of patentability (novelty, inventive step, and industrial applicability) and a uniform patent term of twenty years. Developing countries were bound to fully implement their TRIPS obligations, including pharmaceutical patents, no later than January 1, 2005. Countries defined as least-developed countries (LDCs) by the United Nations had at least until January 1, 2006 to implement TRIPS obligations. For pharmaceutical patents and test data protection, the Doha Declaration (see below) extended this transition period until 2016. Therefore, LDCs do not have to grant or enforce local patents until January 1, 2016 with a possibility of further extension.

The TRIPS Agreement attempts to strike a balance between the interests of right holders and users and contains elements of flexibility to pursue public policy goals such as the protection of public health. Apart from disclosure of the invention as the fundamental obligation of a patent owner, the most important provisions are: exceptions from the requirement of patentability; research exceptions; compulsory licensing (see Topic 11.1); and freedom to provide for international exhaustion (see Topic 11.3). For compulsory licenses, Article 31 of the TRIPS Agreement establishes various conditions, aimed at protecting legitimate interests of the patent holder. However, TRIPS places no restrictions on the grounds on which such licenses may be granted.

To affirm and enhance flexibilities contained in the TRIPS Agreement, WTO Members adopted the "*Declaration on the TRIPS Agreement and Public Health*" at the Doha WTO Ministerial Conference in November 2001. The Doha Declaration stresses that the TRIPS Agreement "can and should be interpreted and implemented in a manner supportive of WTO Members' right to protect public health and, in particular, to promote access to medicines for all" and underscores existing room for that in the Agreement.

An issue left unresolved by the Doha Declaration was how to ensure access to medicines in countries with insufficient or no capacity to manufacture the product in question. In 2003, a waiver was adopted at the WTO to overcome the limitation anchored in TRIPS that compulsory licenses must be authorized predominantly for the supply of the domestic market of the member granting the license. The system established under the waiver decision essentially requires the granting of a compulsory license in the exporting country and imposes notification requirements on the importing country (plus a compulsory license if the product is on patent in that country). The waiver decision establishes various other conditions as well. In December 2005, the waiver decision was transformed into a permanent amendment of the TRIPS Agreement, currently awaiting ratification by WTO members.

Practice Examples

In 2005, India, a key supplier of generic ARVs to developing countries, amended its patent law to conform to the TRIPS Agreement, thereby ushering in a new era of Indian pharmaceutical product patents and raising global concern about the future supply of low-cost ARVs to developing countries. The Patents (Amendment) Act, 2005 can be found, together with a wealth of related material, at http://www.cptech.org/ip/health/c/india/ (Provision Section 92A gives effect to the 2003 WTO waiver decision).

Various potential exporting countries (including Canada, China, the EU, India, the Netherlands, and Norway) have implemented the 2003 WTO waiver decision in their legislation, but the system established by the decision has not yet been used.

In Canada, the so-called *Jean Chrétien Pledge to Africa Act* was the first such effort at reform. It amends the Patent Act by adding a section on "Use of Patents for International Humanitarian Purposes to Address Public Health Problems." The purpose of this amendment is "facilitating access to pharmaceutical products to address public health problems afflicting many developing and least-developed countries, especially those resulting from HIV/AIDS, tuberculosis, malaria and other epidemics." It is available, together with extensive commentary by the Canadian HIV/AIDS Legal Network, at http://www.aidslaw.ca and at http://camr-rcam.hc-sc.gc.ca/index_e.html

The Netherlands' rules of Dec. 21, 2004, EC Regulation No. 816/2006 and information on various other implementing legislative schemes are available at http://www.cptech.org/ip/health/cl/cl-export-legislation.html

Aside from the major report of the Commission on Intellectual Property Rights, Innovation and Public Health cited below, the World Health Organization has published a number of papers and reports on the subject. See in the references, for example, Carlos M. Correa (2002, 2004); German Velasquez & Jaume Vidal (2003); Médecins sans Frontières (2004). The website of the Consumer Project on Technology has a rich collection of information and materials. (http://www.cptech.org/ip/health)

References

Abbott, Frederick M., *The WTO Medicines Decision: World Pharmaceutical Trade and the Protection of Public Health,* 99(2) Am. J. of Int'l Law 317–58 (2005).

Abbott, Frederick M. & Rudolf V. van Puymbroeck, *Compulsory Licensing for Public Health: A Guide and Model Documents for Implementation of the Doha Declaration Paragraph 6 Decision,* 61 World Bank Working Paper (World Bank 2005).

Correa, Carlos M., *Implications of the Doha Declaration on the TRIPS Agreement and Public Health,* EDM Series 12 (World Health Organization 2002).

Correa, Carlos M., *Implementation of the WTO General Council Decision on Paragraph 6 of the Doha Declaration on the TRIPS Agreement and Public Health,* EDM Series 16 (World Health Organization 2004).

European Union, *Regulation (EC) No 816/2006 of the European Parliament and of the Council of 17 May 2006 on Compulsory Licensing of Patents Relating to the Manufacture of Pharmaceutical Products for Export to Countries with Public Health Problems,* 157(1) OJ EU L (2006). http://eur-lex.europa.eu/LexUriServ/site/en/oj/2006/l_157/l_15720060609en00010007.pdf

Fink, Carsten, *Intellectual Property and Public Health: The WTO's August 2003 Decision in Perspective,* in *Trade, Doha, and Development: A Window on the Issues* (Richard Newfarmer, ed., World Bank 2006). http://siteresources.worldbank.org/INTRANETTRADE/Resources/239054-1126812419270/15.PublicHealth.pdf

Gamharter, Katharina, *Access to Affordable Medicines: Developing Responses under the TRIPS Agreement and EC Law,* Europainstitut Wirtschaftsuniversität Wien Publication Series 25 (Springer 2004).

Health Systems Resource Centre, DfID, *Access to Medicines in Under-Served Markets: What Are the Implications of Changes in Intellectual Property Rights, Trade, and Drug Registration Policy?* (Health Systems Resource Centre, Department for International Development 2004). http://www.dfidhealthrc.org/

Médecins sans Frontières, *Determining the Patent Status of Essential Medicines in Developing Countries,* EDM Series 17 (World Health Organization 2004).

Velasquez, German & Jaume Vidal, *IPR, Innovation, Human Rights and Access to Drugs: An Annotated Bibliography,* EDM Series 14 (3rd ed., World Health Organization 2003).

WHO, *Public Health, Innovation, and Intellectual Property Rights: Report of the Commission on Intellectual Property Rights, Innovation, and Public Health* (World Health Organization 2006). http://www.who.int/intellectualproperty/documents/thereport/ CIPIHReport23032006.pdf

WTO, *TRIPS and Public Health* (World Trade Organization, accessed 04/13/2007). http://www.wto.org/english/tratop_e/trips_e/pharmpatent_e.htm

11.3 Parallel Importing, Exhaustion of Patent Rights, Differential Pricing

The Issue

Patented drugs sell at different prices in different national or regional markets. If a procurement authority in country B finds a patented drug for a cheaper price in country A, can it be imported legally?

Legal and Policy Considerations

If drugs that the patent holder has placed on the market in market A are imported into market B without the consent of the patent holder, this is referred to as "parallel importing." It is important to note that this applies only to products legitimately put on the market by the patent holder and not to counterfeit goods or illegal copies.

Whether "parallel importing" is legal depends on how the question of so-called patent "exhaustion" is dealt with under the importing country's legal system. "Exhaustion" refers to the loss of the right to control the resale of the protected product after the first sale by means of an intellectual property right (here, a patent). Three types of exhaustion can be distinguished: national, regional, and international. Within a national market, the right is exhausted as soon as the product is put on the market by a right holder or with his consent. Subsequent resale *within* the country can no longer be controlled. However, under national exhaustion, the holder of a patent retains the right to control the resale of the product in national market B if the product has been sold with his consent in national market A. Therefore, he may prevent parallel importing from market A into market B.

Under regional exhaustion, the effect of national exhaustion is extended to a group of two or more countries. Therefore, the sale in any of the participating countries exhausts the right to control the resale within the entire region. International exhaustion expands this concept to a global scale. As a consequence, under our example, if the product has been sold with the consent of the patent holder in national market A, this sale exhausts the patent right globally and the patent holder can no longer prevent parallel imports by third parties into country B.

An important clarification of the Doha Declaration (see Topic 11.2) was that WTO Members are free under the TRIPS Agreement to adopt the exhaustion regime that best fits their needs—this means that countries are free to allow parallel importing. However, the role of parallel imports as a sustainable source of low-priced medicines is disputed. Points of caution include that the control of drug quality may be more complicated if drugs are not directly procured from the patent holder, and that parallel importing limits the application of differential pricing.

Differential or equity pricing provides for lower prices for medicines in developing countries. Differential pricing refers to the adaptation of prices charged by the patent owner to the purchasing power of governments and households in different countries. Underlying economic theory suggests that prices should be inversely related to price sensitivity in each market, which would lead to lower prices in the markets of developing countries. Differential pricing relies on the possibility of international market segmentation and, therefore, parallel importation can undermine equity or differential pricing.

Practice Examples

The Kenyan *Industrial Property Act 2001* currently incorporates an international exhaustion regime. Section 58(2) provides:

> "The rights under the patent shall not extend to acts in respect of articles which have been put on the market in Kenya or in any other country or imported into Kenya."

While this is a particularly broad formulation, it is in line with the flexibilities available under the TRIPS Agreement.

In order to promote differential pricing by pharmaceutical producers rather than parallel importation, the EU has adopted *Regulation 953/2003*. This regulation establishes an import ban into the EU for pharmaceuticals related to HIV and AIDS, malaria and tuberculosis sold at preferential prices in developing countries, if procedures as established in the Regulation are followed.

References

Commission on Intellectual Property Rights, *Integrating Intellectual Property Rights and Development Policy: Report of the Commission on Intellectual Property Rights* (Commission on Intellectual Property Rights 2002). http://www.iprcommission.org/graphic/documents/final_report.htm

European Union, *Regulation (EC) No 816/2006 of the European Parliament and of the Council of 17 May 2006 on Compulsory Licensing of Patents Relating to the Manufacture of Pharmaceutical Products for Export to Countries with Public Health Problems*, 157(1) OJ EU L (2006). http://eur-lex.europa.eu/LexUriServ/site/en/oj/2006/l_157/l_15720060609en00010007.pdf

Musungu, Sisule F. & Cecilia Oh, *The Use of Flexibilities in TRIPS by Developing Countries: Can They Promote Access to Medicines,* Case Study 4C, August (Commission on Intellectual Property Rights, Innovation, and Public Health, World Health Organization 2005). http://www.who.int/intellectualproperty/studies/TRIPS_flexibilities/en/index.html

WHO, *Public Health, Innovation, and Intellectual Property Rights: Report of the Commission on Intellectual Property Rights, Innovation, and Public Health* (World Health Organization 2006). http://www.who.int/intellectualproperty/documents/thereport/CIPIHReport 23032006.pdf

11.4   Free Trade Agreements: Special Considerations

The Issue

Regional and bilateral free trade agreements (FTAs), particularly as concluded by the United States, commonly include commitments in the area of intellectual property rights. Frequently these go beyond what is required by the TRIPS Agreement and the Doha Declaration (see Topic 11.2). These stricter, so-called "TRIPS-plus" provisions undermine the flexibilities countries have under TRIPS and may impair access to medicines.

Legal and Policy Considerations

The U.S. pursues an active regional and bilateral free trade agreements program (e.g., the *Central America-Dominican Republic-United States Free Trade Agreement,* or CAFTA-DR, and the FTAs with Jordan, Singapore, Chile, Australia, Morocco, Colombia, and Peru). These agreements aim at comprehensive trade opening to enhance economic growth and welfare. However, the provisions on market access tend to be accompanied by commitments on intellectual property rights, including patents. These provisions frequently go beyond what is required by the TRIPS Agreement and the Doha Declaration. It is important, therefore, always to check the text of any FTAs to which a country is a party. U.S. trade agreements: http://www.ustr.gov/Trade_Agreements/Section_Index.html.

TRIPS-plus provisions in regional and bilateral FTAs have included: possible extensions of the patent term, more stringent protection of pharmaceutical test data than required by Art. 39.3 of the TRIPS Agreement, and establishment of a linkage between marketing approval (drug registration) and patent status. Other limitations of TRIPS flexibilities include restrictions on the grounds for compulsory licensing, expansion of patent scope and limits to challenging potentially invalid patents.

Accompanying some of these FTAs are side letters that appear to indicate that the agreement's intellectual property requirements do not affect the other party's ability to take necessary measures to protect public health and the promotion of access to medicines for all. However, the interpretation and legal enforceability of these side letters is unclear.

Practice Example

Article 15.10(2) of the CAFTA-DR provides:

"2. Where a Party permits, as a condition of approving the marketing of a pharmaceutical product, persons, other than the person originally submitting safety or efficacy information, to rely on evidence or information concerning the safety and efficacy of a product that was previously approved, such as evidence of prior marketing approval in the territory of a Party or in another country, that Party:

(a) shall implement measures in its marketing approval process to prevent such other persons from marketing a product covered by a patent claiming the previously approved product or its approved use during the term of that patent, unless by consent or acquiescence of the patent owner; and

(b) shall provide that the patent owner shall be informed of the request and the identity of any such other person who requests approval to enter the market during the term of a patent identified as claiming the approved product or its approved use."

This provision links marketing approval for generics to the patent status of the originator product. As a consequence, marketing approval (or registration) for generics cannot be obtained during the patent term, except with the consent or acquiescence of the patent owner. This goes beyond both the requirements for patent and for test data protection as established in the TRIPS Agreement, may preclude the use of compulsory licenses, and may result in reduced access to HIV medications in countries party to these agreements.

References

Commission on Intellectual Property Rights, *Integrating Intellectual Property Rights and Development Policy, Report of the Commission on Intellectual Property Rights* (Commission on Intellectual Property Rights 2002). http://www.iprcommission.org/graphic/documents/final_report.htm

Fink, Carsten & Patrick Reichenmiller, *Tightening TRIPS: Intellectual Property Provisions of U.S. Free Trade Agreements,* in *Trade, Doha, and Development: A Window on the Issues* (Richard Newfarmer, ed., World Bank 2006). http://siteresources.worldbank.org/INTRANETTRADE/Resources/239054-1126812419270/24.TighteningTRIPS.pdf

Jorge, Maria Fabiana, *TRIPS-Plus Provisions in Trade Agreements and Their Potential Adverse Effects on Public Health,* 3(April) Journal of Generic Medicines (2004).

Musungu, Sisule F. & Cecilia Oh, *Bilateral and Regional FTAs: Practical Implications for Access to Medicines in Developing Countries,* Chapter IV in *The Use of Flexibilities in TRIPS by Developing Countries: Can They Promote Access to Medicines*, Case Study 4C, August (Commission on Intellectual Property Rights, Innovation, and Public Health, World Health Organization 2005). http://www.who.int/intellectualproperty/studies/TRIPS_flexibilities/en/index.html

WHO, *Public Health, Innovation and Intellectual Property Rights: Report of the Commission on Intellectual Property Rights, Innovation and Public Health* (World Health Organization 2006). http://www.who.int/intellectualproperty/documents/thereport/CIPIHReport23032006.pdf

World Bank Policies and Procedures

12.1   IDA Grants for HIV and AIDS Projects

The Issue

Most international financing for HIV/AIDS projects is now on grant terms. Under the Thirteenth Replenishment of the resources of IDA (IDA 13), HIV/AIDS projects benefited from an exception to regular IDA terms and received 100 percent grant financing in IDA-only countries and up to 25 percent grant financing in blend countries.[1] Under the terms of the Fourteenth Replenishment (IDA 14) for the period FY06–08, this special rule for HIV/AIDS projects no longer applies. Based on the application of criteria relating to debt vulnerability, IDA-only countries may now qualify for grant financing for 100 or 50 percent of their total allocation. Some IDA-only countries only receive standard IDA credit terms.

Legal and Policy Considerations

Under the IDA 14 arrangements, grant financing is:

- Limited to IDA-only countries; and
- Based on a country-by-country analysis of the risk of debt distress.

The following provisions apply:

- Countries that are reclassified from blend country to IDA-only country prior to the IDA 14 mid-term review will continue to be ineligible for grants over the entire course of IDA 14.
- As an exception to the debt distress-based rule for grant eligibility, both Kosovo and Timor Leste benefit from grant terms. However, Timor Leste will be gradually phased out of grant eligibility over the IDA 14 period.
- IDA may finance on a grant basis the portion of the cost of regional projects attributable to IDA-only countries eligible for 100 percent grants under the debt-distress criterion.

In application of these provisions, HIV/AIDS projects may thus continue to benefit from grant terms in certain countries.

---

[1] The International Development Association (IDA) provides interest-free loans, called credits, to governments of the poorest countries. The World Bank lends to governments of middle-income and creditworthy low-income countries. "Blend countries" are eligible to receive a combination of Bank loans and IDA credits. A list of countries by category is available at http://www.worldbank.org.

For FY07 (July 1, 2006 to June 30, 2007) a 100 percent IDA grant allocation applies to: Afghanistan, Bhutan, Burundi, Cambodia, Central African Republic, Chad, Comoros, Congo (Democratic Republic of), Congo (Republic of), Cote d'Ivoire, Djibouti, Eritrea, The Gambia, Guinea, Guinea-Bissau, Haiti, Kosovo, Kyrgyz Republic, Lao PDR, Liberia, Myanmar, Nepal, Niger, Rwanda, Sao Tome and Principe, Sierra Leone, Solomon Islands, Somalia, Sudan, Togo, and Tonga. For FY07 a 50 percent IDA grant allocation applies to: Angola, Ethiopia, Guyana, Lesotho, Malawi, Mongolia, Nicaragua, Samoa, Sri Lanka, Tajikistan. Timor Leste is eligible for a 60 percent IDA grant allocation, phasing down to 30% in FY08.

Grant-eligible countries for subsequent fiscal years will be listed in Operational Policy (OP) 3.10, Annex D—IBRD/IDA Countries: Per Capita Incomes, Lending Eligibility, and Repayment Terms, which is updated annually.

Practice Examples

An IDA grant in the amount of SDR 99.3 million was approved for the Democratic Republic of Congo Health Sector Rehabilitation Support Project on September 1, 2005.

An IDA credit of SDR 13.7 million on standard IDA terms was approved for the Ghana Multi-Sectoral HIV/AIDS Project on November 15, 2005.

References

World Bank, *Additions to IDA Resources: Thirteenth Replenishment,* IDA/SecM2002-0488, Sept. 17 (World Bank 2002). http://siteresources.worldbank.org/IDA/Resources/FinaltextIDA13Report.pdf

————, *Additions to IDA Resources: Fourteenth Replenishment,* IDA/R2005-0029 (World Bank 2005). http://siteresources.worldbank.org/IDA/Resources/14th_Replenishment_Final.pdf

————, *Debt Sustainability and Financing Terms in IDA 14: Further Considerations on Issues and Options* (World Bank 2004). http://siteresources.worldbank.org/IDA/Resources/DebtSustainabilityNov04.pdf

————, *IBRD/IDA Countries: Per Capita Incomes, Lending Eligibility, and Repayment Terms,* OP 3.10, Annex D (World Bank 2005). http://intranet.worldbank.org/WBSITE/INTRANET/OPSMANUAL/0,,pagePK:60000988~theSitePK:210385,00.html

————, *Implementing the IDA14 Resource Allocation Framework in FY07* (Resource Mobilization Department, World Bank 2006). http://intresources.worldbank.org/INTCFP/Resources/IDA14AllocationImplementationFY07.pdf

12.2   OP/BP 4.01 and Medical Waste Management

The Issue

All projects proposed for World Bank financing are screened for environmental impact. Depending on the type, location, sensitivity, and scale of the project and the nature and magnitude of its potential environmental impacts, proposed projects are assigned a classification that determines the further actions to be taken, if any, to reduce and manage risks associated with the project. These measures are spelled out in Operational Policy/Bank Procedure (OP/BP) 4.01.

HIV/AIDS projects typically include prevention, care and treatment and mitigation activities. Some of these activities lead to waste products (including infectious and pathological waste) that can pose serious threats to health workers and communities if not properly handled and disposed of. In addition to health care waste management of HIV-specific activities, projects may also finance the strengthening of medical and biomedical waste management systems in public health facilities more generally.

Legal and Policy Considerations

Environmental assessment of the waste management issues in HIV/AIDS projects typically triggers a Category B classification under OP 4.01. The OP and its accompanying BP detail the actions to be taken (a) by the Borrower with respect to the preparation of safeguard documents (such as risk assessments and management plans), public consultation, disclosure, compliance, and monitoring and progress reporting; and (b) by the Bank in processing the project. In countries with health care waste management systems that reflect the objectives and operational principles of OP/BP 4.01, under the provisions of OP 4.00, the Bank may simply authorize the application of existing country systems for Bank funded projects.

The legal documents for the project must include one or more covenants recording the Borrower's commitment to implement medical waste management plans approved by the Bank and ensuring applicability of the Bank's remedies in case of noncompliance. The Bank does not finance project activities that would contravene the country's obligations under international agreements as identified during the environmental assessment (OP 4.01, para. 3). The relevant conventions are: the *Stockholm Convention on Persistent Organic Pollutants* (POPs) and the *Basel Convention on the Control of Transboundary Movements of Hazardous Wastes and Their Disposal*.

Practice Example

Development Grant Agreement (Multi-Sectoral HIV/AIDS Project) between the Republic of Malawi and the International Development Association dated September 11, 2003 (IDA Grant No. H062 MAI):

> "'Health Care Waste Management Plan' or 'HCWMP' means the Recipient's plan dated July 4, 2003, setting out the measures to be undertaken to ensure proper management of hazardous waste under the Project" (Art. I, Section 1.01 (m)).

> "The Recipient shall cause NAC to: (i) prepare and furnish to the Association an Operational Manual, in form and substance satisfactory to the Association; (ii) implement the Project in accordance with the arrangements and procedures set out in the Memorandum of Understanding, the Operational Manual, and the Health Care Waste Management Plan; and (iii) except as the Association shall otherwise agree, not amend, abrogate or waive any provision thereof which may, in the opinion of the Association, materially and adversely affect the implementation of the Project." (Schedule 4, Implementation Program, Section I, paragraph 3).

> "Without limitation upon the provisions of Section I of this Schedule, the Recipient shall cause NAC to appraise, approve, coordinate, monitor and evaluate Subprograms under Parts 1 through 6 of Schedule 2 to this Agreement, and administer Subprogram Grants, in accordance with the provisions and procedures set forth in this Section III and in more detail in the Memorandum of Understanding, the Operational Manual and the Health Care Waste management Plan, and shall not make any material change to any approved Subprogram without consultation and approval of the Association." (Schedule 4, Implementation Program, Section III, paragraph 1 (a)).

References

Brown, Jonathan C., Didem Ayvalikli & Nadeem Mohammed, *Medical Waste Management*, Chapter 6 in *Turning Bureaucrats into Warriors: Preparing and Implementing Multi-Sector HIV-AIDS Programs in Africa, a Generic Operations Manual* (World Bank 2004). http://www.worldbank.org/afr/aids

WHO, *Safe Management of Wastes from Health-Care Activities* (World Health Organization 1999). http://www.healthcarewaste.org. See especially Chapter 2, *Definition and Characterization of Health Care Waste*, and Chapter 4, *Legislative, Regulatory, and Policy Aspects*.

World Bank, *Health Care Waste Management* (World Bank 2003). http://web.worldbank.org/phataglance

12.3   OP/BP 4.10 and Indigenous Peoples in HIV and AIDS Projects

The Issue

Indigenous people tend to be disproportionately affected by HIV due to a variety of factors: social marginalization, poverty, gender, traditional intergenerational relations, and isolation from sources of information and services, all can play a role in contributing to the ultimate impact of HIV in the population.

HIV/AIDS projects, either standing alone or as part of national or regional programs to strengthen the health sector, may finance prevention, care, support, and treatment activities in areas where indigenous people are present. In such cases, special care needs to be taken to ensure that these people's dignity, human rights, economies, and cultures are fully respected.

Legal and Policy Considerations

All projects proposed for World Bank financing that affect indigenous peoples must comply with the requirements of Operational Policy/Bank Procedure (OP/BP) 4.10—Indigenous Peoples. In essence, OP/BP 4.10 requires: a screening by the Bank to ascertain whether indigenous peoples are present in, or have a collective attachment to, the project area; a social assessment by the Borrower; a process of free, prior and informed consultation with the affected communities at each stage of the project and ascertainment of broad community support for the project; the preparation of an indigenous peoples plan or planning framework, which must be available for the Bank's review prior to appraisal; and public disclosure of the plan or planning framework. The detailed requirements are set out in the OP/BP and Annexes.

The legal documents for the project must ensure that the indigenous peoples plan or planning framework is in place by the time of loan/credit/grant effectiveness, and must provide for the applicability of the Bank's legal remedies in case of noncompliance.

Practice Example

Loan Agreement (Third AIDS and STD Control Project) between the Federative Republic of Brazil and the International Bank for Reconstruction and Development dated November 27, 2003 (Loan No. 4713-BR):

> "'Indigenous Peoples Action Plan' means the Borrower's plan for benefiting indigenous peoples under the Project as set forth in the document furnished by MOH to the Bank on June 3, 2003" (Art. I, Section 1.01 (u)).

"The Borrower shall, through MOH, enter into an agreement with FUNASA under terms and conditions satisfactory to the Bank, setting forth in respect of the Indigenous Peoples Action Plan, *inter alia,* FUNASA's obligation to participate in its implementation and provide the required counterpart funding" (Art. III, Section 3.01 (e)).

"The Borrower shall carry out the Project in accordance with an operational manual, satisfactory to the Bank, said manual to include, *inter alia*: . . . the Indigenous Peoples Action Plan" (Art. III, Section 3.03 (e)).

"The Borrower shall, through MOH, carry out and cause FUNASA to carry out the Indigenous Peoples Action Plan in accordance with its terms" (Art. III, Section 3.05).

References

UNAIDS & OHCHR, *International Guidelines on HIV/AIDS and Human Rights,* 2006 Consolidated version, paragraph 97 (UNAIDS & Office of the United Nations High Commissioner for Human Rights 2006). http://data.unaids.org/Publications/IRC-pub07/JC1252-InternGuidelines_en.pdf?preview=true

World Bank, *Project Appraisal Document on a Proposed Loan in the Amount of US$100.00 Million to the Federative Republic of Brazil for the AIDS & STD Control III Project* (World Bank 2003). http://www-wds.worldbank.org/servlet/WDS_IBank_Servlet?pcont=details&eid=000094946_03040104042918

———, *Social Assessment, Indigenous Peoples Development Plan,* Annex 2(c) in *Project Appraisal Document on a Proposed Loan in the Amount of US$100.00 Million to the Federative Republic of Brazil for the AIDS & STD Control III Project* (World Bank 2003). http://www-wds.worldbank.org/servlet/WDS_IBank_Servlet?pcont=details&eid=000094946_03040104042918

———, *Indigenous Peoples,* Operational Manual, OP/BP 4.10 (World Bank 2005). http://wbln0018.worldbank.org/Institutional/Manuals/OpManual.nsf/B52929624EB2A3538525672E00775F66/DBB9575225027E678525703100541C7D?OpenDocument. See Annex A, *Social Assessment*; Annex B, *Indigenous Peoples Plan*; and Annex C, *Indigenous Peoples Planning Framework.*

12.4 Communities and CBOs: Fiduciary Issues

The Issue

Projects financed under the Multi-Country AIDS Program (MAP) for Africa and other similar Bank-supported projects provide funds to communities and community-based organizations (CBOs) in order to support grass-roots responses to the epidemic. Communities and CBOs differ from NGOs and other civil society organizations in that they tend to be less formally organized, and sometimes may not have any formal structure at all. This raises special challenges with respect to the Bank's fiduciary obligations concerning financial management, procurement, and disbursement.

Legal and Policy Considerations

Unless required under the laws of the country, the Bank does not require official registration or incorporation of communities and CBOs as a condition for access to World Bank funds through a MAP-type project.

Operational policies on financial management (OP 10.02), procurement (OP 11.00), and disbursement (OP 12.00) apply to all Bank-financed projects. Because of special considerations relating to management capacity and the scale of operations, further guidance on the implementation of these policies has been developed for community-driven development projects. This guidance is also applicable to community- or CBO-executed activities under MAP or other World Bank-financed AIDS loans, credits or grants.

Procurement, disbursement, and financial management by communities should follow the guidance provided in the document *Fiduciary Management for Community-Driven Development Projects: A Reference Guide* prepared by the Procurement and Financial Management Sector Boards.

In implementation of Operational Policy 11.00 and the above-mentioned Reference Guide, further practical guidance on procurement by CBOs under Africa MAP projects is provided in the document *Generic Procurement Management Manual for Community Based Organizations and Local NGOs* prepared by the ACT*Africa* group. This manual is useful also for procurement by CBOs generally, and not just in Africa MAP projects.

Clear and practical information on implementation of Operational Policy 12.00 (Disbursement) is available in *World Bank HIV/AIDS Program: A Guidance Note on Disbursement Procedures* prepared by the Bank's Loan Department. Section III of this Guidance Note deals with funding procedures for community-level implementing organizations.

Practice Example

Development Credit Agreement between Republic of Burundi and International Development Association (Multisectoral HIV/AIDS Control and Orphans Project) dated July 25, 2002 (Credit No. 3684 BU):

"6. Community Participation
Goods and works required for CSO Subprojects shall be procured in accordance with procedures acceptable to the Association and defined in the Project Implementation Manual" (Schedule 3, Section I, Part C.6).

"'CSO' means a civil society organization established and operating under the laws of the Borrower, including rural or urban communities, grass-root organizations, religious and cultural organizations, professional and non-professional associations, private enterprises, NGOs and community-based associations involved in the fight against HIV/AIDS and which have met the eligibility criteria set out in the Project Implementation Manual and the requirements of Schedule 4 to this Agreement and, as a result, have received or are entitled to receive a grant . . . for the carrying out of a CSO Subproject . . ." (Article I, Section 1.01 (m)).

Detailed provisions for CSO Subprojects are set out in Schedule 4 (Implementation Program), Section 4.

References

Brown, Jonathan C., Didem Ayvalikli & Nadeem Mohammad, *Turning Bureaucrats into Warriors: Preparing and Implementing Multi-Sector HIV-AIDS Programs in Africa, a Generic Operations Manual* (World Bank 2004). http://www.worldbank.org/afr/aids

World Bank, *Fiduciary Management for Community-Driven Development Projects: A Reference Guide* (World Bank 2002). http://siteresources.worldbank.org/INTAFRREGTOPHIVAIDS/Resources/03Fiduciary-Mng-for-CDD.pdf

————, *Generic Procurement Management Manual for Community Based Organizations and Local NGOs* (World Bank 2003). http://siteresources.worldbank.org/INTAFRREGTOPHIVAIDS/Resources/01CBO-Procurement-Manual-English.pdf

————, *HIV/AIDS Program: A Guidance Note on Disbursement Procedures* (World Bank 2005). http://siteresources.worldbank.org/INTHIVAIDS/Resources/375798-1098987393985/HIVAIDSGuidanceNoteonDisbProcedures.pdf

12.5   Procurement of Pharmaceutical Products

The Issue

Other than questions relating to patents and international agreements dealt with in Chapter 11 on procurement of antiretroviral medicines (ARVs), other medicines required in the care of people with HIV, and related products (such as testing kits) may pose special issues as a result of national regulatory requirements, restricted sources of supply, or the government's participation in the Clinton Foundation's procurement scheme.

Legal and Policy Considerations

The law of most countries provides that only pharmaceutical products approved by the national drug regulatory authority (frequently referred to as "registered" drugs) may be imported into or sold within the country. Consequently, suppliers of pharmaceutical products should always be required to demonstrate compliance with national registration requirements as a condition for contract effectiveness. Countries may provide a fast-track registration process for certain types of drugs (life-saving drugs, unique drugs for which no alternatives exist, or well-established generics).

Because the national drug regulatory authorities of many countries have limited technical capacity, the Bank's prequalification requirements will typically include the condition that the product be prequalified under the WHO-administered United Nations Procurement Quality and Sourcing Project, or authorized under the Pharmaceutical Inspection Convention, the Pharmaceutical Inspection Cooperation Scheme, or the International Conference on Harmonization of Technical Requirements for the Registration of Pharmaceuticals for Human Use. (Pharmaceutical Inspection Convention and Pharmaceutical Inspection Cooperation Scheme: http://www.picscheme.org/index.htm and International Conference on Harmonization of Technical Requirements for the Registration of Pharmaceuticals for Human Use: http://www.ich.org)

Due to supply limitations resulting from patents and registration requirements, many ARVs and related products are single-source or limited source products for procurement purposes. International or national competitive bidding, with or without prequalification, is, therefore, not the rule. Depending on the circumstances, limited international bidding, shopping, direct contracting or procurement through specialized UN agencies, may be the indicated procurement methods. Detailed guidance is provided in the procurement chapter of Taylor (2004).

Under the HIV/AIDS initiative of the William J. Clinton Foundation, low- and middle-income countries may be able to procure key antiretroviral medicines, including pediatric formulations, and diagnostic tests at or below prices published by the Foundation, which in turn are significantly lower than market prices. The Clinton Foundation is able to obtain suppliers' commitments to these prices on the basis of a set of operating principles that include volume discounts, medium to long term contracts, splitting of orders among suppliers, and payment upon shipment. Some of these principles are inconsistent with standard World Bank procurement rules. Hence, in order to enable borrowing member countries to take advantage of the economies offered by the Clinton Foundation's procurement scheme, modifications to the Standard Bidding Documents have been adopted and are available on the OPCPR website ("Modifications to SBD Health Sector Goods to Accommodate Clinton Foundation Requirements"). Staff should also follow "Instructions to Staff—Collaboration with the Clinton Foundation," also available on the website of OPCPR, which provides further helpful information and instructions. It should be noted that under World Bank-financed procurements with accommodations for the Clinton Foundation scheme, competitive bidding is still required and any prequalified bidder must be allowed to bid regardless of whether the bidder is a member of the Clinton Foundation Procurement Consortium. (Clinton Foundation HIV/AIDS Initiative: http://www.clintonfoundation.org)

Practice Example

The Clinton Foundation signed a memorandum of understanding with the Dominican Republic for the application of its procurement scheme. The legal document for the restructuring of the World Bank-supported HIV/AIDS Prevention and Control Project of the Dominican Republic includes the following procurement paragraph:

> "Procurement methods for medicines, specialized medical supplies and laboratory equipment (e.g., vaccines, antituberculosis drugs, antiretroviral drugs, condoms, test kits, reagents, viral load and CD count machines) will be determined by the Borrower, subject to the Bank's no-objection, taking into account the market situation of each product (i.e., the number of available qualified suppliers and other relevant considerations pertaining to the product in question). Subject to the foregoing, they may be procured, regardless of the contract value, using Limited International Bidding (LIB), shopping or Direct Contracting procedures in accordance with the provisions of paragraphs 3.2, 3.5, 3.6, and 3.9 [of the Procurement Guidelines]."

References

World Bank, *Standard Bidding Documents, Procurement of Health Sector Goods (Pharmaceuticals, Vaccines, and Condoms)* (World Bank 2004). http://web.worldbank.org/WBSITE/EXTERNAL/PROJECTS/PROCUREMENT/0,,contentMDK:20199935~menuPK:84284~pagePK:84269~piPK:60001558~theSitePK:84266,00.html

―――, *Modifications to SBD Health Sector Goods to Accommodate Clinton Foundation Requirements* (World Bank 2004). http://web.worldbank.org/WBSITE/EXTERNAL/PROJECTS/PROCUREMENT/0,,contentMDK:20199935~menuPK:84284~pagePK:84269~piPK:60001558~theSitePK:84266,00.html

―――, *Instructions to Staff: Collaboration with the Clinton Foundation* (World Bank 2004). http://web.worldbank.org/WBSITE/EXTERNAL/PROJECTS/PROCUREMENT/0,,contentMDK:50002392~menuPK:93977~pagePK:84269~piPK:60001558~theSitePK:84266,00.html

Taylor, Yolanda, ed., *Battling HIV/AIDS: A Decision-Maker's Guide to the Procurement of Medicines and Related Supplies,* Chapter 2 in *Intellectual Property Rights: A Concise Guide* (World Bank 2004). www.worldbank.org/aids

World Bank, *Procurement of Health Sector Goods,* Technical Note, May (World Bank 2000, revised 2006). http://web.worldbank.org/WBSITE/EXTERNAL/PROJECTS/PROCUREMENT/0,,contentMDK:20199935~menuPK:84284~pagePK:84269~piPK:60001558~theSitePK:84266,00.html

12.6 Procurement of Condoms

The Issue

Condoms must be of high quality to have their intended prophylactic effect, and production is technically demanding. While there are many manufacturers, relatively few companies are responsible for most international sales. As an alternative to purchasing directly from the manufacturer or supplier, condoms may be procured from or through UNFPA and other UN agencies (such as UNDP's Inter-Agency Procurement Services Office, IAPSO) offering relevant procurement services.

Distribution to target groups may require merchandising expertise not available locally. It can be furnished by specialized service providers, including social marketing enterprises, in which case the marketing services are bundled with the supply of condoms. Social marketing of condoms combines commercial sales techniques with the promotion of healthier behaviors.

Legal and Policy Considerations

The Bank strongly supports prequalification of condom suppliers. The Standard Bidding Documents for Procurement of Health Sector Goods contain provisions for condom procurement in the Special Conditions of Contract (Inspections and Tests; Delivery and Documents) and in the Sample Technical Specifications.

Condoms are considered a multisource product and large purchases are therefore typically handled under International Competitive Bidding (ICB). Specialized UN agencies may be used as direct suppliers under paragraph 3.9 of the *Procurement Guidelines* (May 2004 edition) or as procurement agents pursuant to paragraph 3.10 of the *Procurement Guidelines* (May 2004 edition), in which case they are hired as consultants pursuant to paragraph 3.15 of the *Consultant Guidelines* (May 2004 edition).

Social marketing enterprises selling condoms are hired under procedures explained in the *Consultants Guidelines,* Quality- and Cost-based Selection procedure.

Practice Examples

The Gambia, Participatory Health, Population and Nutrition Project:

- Project Appraisal Document (Rep. No. 17399 GM): Annex 6, Table A1, Component 1.2: Prevention of Unwanted Pregnancies: Social Marketing Program (Int. TA and Nat. TA): QCBS

- Development Credit Agreement, May 15, 1998: "Goods, essential drugs and contraceptives may be procured from IAPSO, UNFPA, UNICEF, WFP, WHO or other UN agency acceptable to the Association, in accordance with the provisions of paragraph 3.9 of the Guidelines" (Schedule 3, Section I, Part C.4).

References

Brown, Jonathan C., Didem Ayvalikli & Nadeem Mohammad, *Turning Bureaucrats into Warriors: A Generic Operations Manual* (World Bank 2004). www.worldbank.or/afr/aids

Merrick, Tom & Joanne Epp, *Condom Procurement Guide* (Population and Reproductive Health Thematic Group, World Bank 2001). http://wbln0018.worldbank.org/HDNet

Tayler, Yolanda, ed., *Battling HIV/AIDS: A Decision Maker's Guide to the Procurement of Medicines and Related Supplies,* Chapter 2 in *Intellectual Property Rights: A Concise Guide* (World Bank 2004). www.worldbank.org/aids

UNAIDS, *Global Directory of Condom Social Marketing Projects and Organizations* (UNAIDS 2001). http://data.unaids.org/Publications/IRC-pub02/JCCondSocMark_en.pdf #search=%22Global%20Directory%20of%20Condom%20Social%20Marketing%20 Projects%20and%20Organizations%22

World Bank, *Standard Bidding Documents, Procurement of Health Sector Goods (Pharmaceuticals, Vaccines, and Condoms)* (World Bank 2004). http://web.worldbank.org/ WBSITE/EXTERNAL/PROJECTS/PROCUREMENT/0,,contentMDK:20199935~menu PK:84284~pagePK:84269~piPK:60001558~theSitePK:84266,00.html

———, *Procurement of Health Sector Goods,* Technical Note, May (World Bank 2000, revised 2006). http://web.worldbank.org/WBSITE/EXTERNAL/PROJECTS/ PROCUREMENT/0,,contentMDK:20199935~menuPK:84284~pagePK:84269~piPK: 60001558~theSitePK:84266,00.html

Index